the
low carb
long term
lifestyle

✴ carolyn humphries

foulsham
LONDON • NEW YORK • TORONTO • SYDNEY

foulsham

The Publishing House, Bennetts Close, Cippenham,
Slough, Berkshire, SL1 5AP, England

ISBN 0-572-02966-7

A CIP record for this book is available from the British Library.

Neither the editors of W. Foulsham & Co. Ltd nor the
author nor the publisher take responsibility for any
possible consequences from any treatment, procedure,
test, exercise, action or application of medication or
preparation by any person reading or following the
information in this book. The publication of this book
does not constitute the practice of medicine, and this
book does not attempt to replace any diet or
instructions from your doctor. The author and
publisher advise the reader to check with a doctor
before administering any medication or undertaking
any course of treatment or exercise.

The nutritional information in this book is based on
data from DEFRA.

Printed in Great Britain by Creative Print and Design (Wales), Ebbw Vale

Contents

Introduction

Low-carbohydrate, high-protein diets are very effective and very popular. The reason is simple: they enable you to lose weight quickly. However, this quick weight loss comes at a heavy price: the foods you are allowed to eat become boring and unpalatable after a while and, worse still, the regime can cause long-term health problems.

This book provides the answer to both these problems. With its innovative diet plan, you will not only achieve quick weight loss at first, but you will also eat appetising, enjoyable meals from day one. The recipes are designed to reflect the delicious style of Mediterranean cooking and they include those high-fat foods we all love. You can still eat butter, cream and olive oils – in moderation – so you won't feel deprived of treats. But in addition, every phase includes the recommended 'five-a-day' helpings of fruit and vegetables, so you'll still be getting plenty of the vitamins and minerals you need.

The plan is divided into four stages, starting with an initial two-week, rapid-weight-loss phase that is planned down to the last detail, giving you mouth-watering recipes for every meal from breakfast to dinner. Phase 2 offers a healthy, satisfying and delicious, long-term eating regime in the form of a pick-and-mix selection of recipes that will allow you to progress gradually and sensibly, towards your desired weight. The third phase then adds in extra carbohydrate 'treats' to make eating and drinking even more enjoyable and the plan ends with Phase 4, which is made up of easy-to-follow guidelines designed to help you maintain the new you. This section is your eating plan for life – but don't be put off by that. The recipes I've put together make up balanced, gourmet main meals that everyone will enjoy, with small portions of carbohydrates, such as rice, pasta or potatoes – so, once you've reached your goal, there is no reason for you to start to gain weight again.

How to Eat Healthily and Still Lose Weight

There are many different weight-reducing diets to choose
from. Some are designed to shed weight quickly, some slowly;
some are intended as a quick fix, other are more long-term.
Whichever type you choose, it is a good idea to learn as much
as possible about the principles of the diet and how it is likely
to affect you. The better you understand how a regime works,
the more likely you are to have success in using it. It is also
important, particularly if you intend to continue to diet for
more than a week or two, that you choose one that gives you
all the nutrition your body needs in order to stay healthy.
Unlike other low-carbohydrate plans, this one does just that.

The principles of a low-carbohydrate diet

A low-carbohydrate diet is a very effective way to achieve
weight loss. It is based on a few very simple principles.

Carbohydrates are the starches and sugars contained in foods
such as breads, cakes, rice, pasta, potatoes, etc. When we eat
carbohydrates our body breaks them down into glucose to use
as energy. If we eat more carbohydrates than our body burns,
they are stored in the body as fat. But if we eat less than our
body requires, the body is forced to burn body fat instead for
energy. This has the effect of reducing our body weight.

To help the body absorb the glucose from the carbohydrates
and turn it into energy, our pancreas produces insulin. The
more starch and sugar we eat, the more insulin is produced.
Insulin also helps the body to store any unused glucose as fat.
If we severely restrict our intake of carbohydrates, the body
reduces its production of insulin and so does not store body fat.

Reducing our intake of carbohydrates is a very efficient way of
losing weight. In addition, once the body is free from large

quantities of carbohydrates, blood sugar levels remain constant and our craving for sugary snacks is reduced, as well as any serious hunger pangs – clearly, a useful aid for dieters.

It is not a good idea to cut out carbohydrates entirely, however. Our bodies do need a small amount of glucose for some vital functions. This may be provided by the intake of a small quantity of carbohydrates or, alternatively, proteins, which can be processed by the liver and turned into sugar.

Ketosis

One of the less attractive side effects of a low-carbohydrate diet is ketosis. This occurs when the liver begins to produce chemicals called ketones, from fatty acids for energy. Any unused ketones cannot be turned back into fat and stored, so are excreted from the body in the urine. Ketosis causes severe bad breath and a metallic taste in the mouth. Some diets encourage such symptoms since they indicate that your body is burning fat. I do not agree and I prefer that ketosis should be avoided. If you start to experience unpleasant symptoms when your carbohydrate intake is very low, eat a small raw carrot or half a red pepper. This will add 4–5 g of carb to your diet. You will still lose weight, although perhaps a little less rapidly. You can do this every time you suffer the symptoms.

Note: Ketosis is not the same thing as ketoacidosis, a dangerous condition that is suffered by people who have diabetes, when the blood pH becomes acutely acidic and blood sugar levels soar. This may occur either because the body is not producing insulin or because it is not using it correctly, so it is not processing sugar for energy. The body then produces ketones for fuel instead.

Healthy eating

Cutting down carbohydrates drastically for a short time for quick weight loss is perfectly acceptable but you should not maintain it for too long or you will become lethargic and ill. Your body needs nutrients from all the food groups to maintain health and vitality, and so any diet – even a weight-reducing one – should include reasonable proportions of all the main food groups given below. The diet plan in this book aims to do this.

PROTEINS

These are used by the body for growth and repair and, when necessary, for energy. The best sources are fish, lean meat, poultry, dairy products, eggs, soya proteins, such as tofu, and Quorn, which is made from a fungus. Pulses – dried peas, beans and lentils – are good sources too, but they are also high in carbohydrates. When on a low-carbohydrate diet, you should eat more proteins than usual in order to maintain the energy levels that your body needs.

CARBOHYDRATES

There are two types of carbohydrate. **Complex carbohydrates** are all the starchy foods such as bread, pasta, rice, cereals (including breakfast cereals) and tubers such as potatoes. **Simple carbohydrates** are sugars and include those naturally found in foods – like fructose in fruit and lactose in milk – as well as refined sugars used in cakes, biscuits (cookies) and sweets (candies). Nutritionally, the starchy ones and the natural sugars in milk, fruit, etc., are usually considered 'good' foods and are used by the body for energy. Refined sugars contain only empty calories – they do not contain any valuable nutrients – and should be avoided.

On a weight-reducing, low-carbohydrate plan, this food group is reduced drastically in the first phase of the diet, but then re-introduced slowly, in limited quantities. The body cannot function properly without carbohydrates in the long term.

VITAMINS AND MINERALS

These are vital for general health and well-being. Many vitamins and minerals are found in fruit and vegetables. Choose fresh, frozen or those that are canned in water or natural juice with no added sugar – and, ideally, no added salt. It is recommended that everyone eat at least five portions a day.

When you begin your low-carb diet, fruit and vegetables have to be very restricted. However, this severely restricted phase is very short, and as you progress through the plan, I introduce lots more variety. It is essential that you eat all those suggested in the diet plan; they are vital to your health. I also recommend you take a good-quality vitamin and mineral supplement daily, although do check that it contains no sugar or starch.

FATS

Like carbohydrates, fats can be converted by the body into energy and are also used for warmth. They are found naturally in foods high in protein – such as dairy products, meat, fish, poultry, nuts, seeds and some fruits, particularly olives and avocados (which makes these a bonus on a low-carb plan).

A low-carbohydrate diet may include some fat – and fat is actually essential for your body to function properly. However, large amounts of animal fats can cause heart problems and strokes, so try not to overdo your intake of butter and cream, and choose lean meats wherever possible.

FIBRE

Fibre is not a food group as such, but it is vital for healthy body functioning. Lack of fibre will make your digestion – and you – sluggish, and may lead to other health problems.

Whilst on your low-carb diet, you should make sure you eat lots of dark green vegetables and lots of nuts and seeds, once these are allowed. Drink plenty of water and take plenty of exercise to help prevent constipation. When you are able to have potatoes and fruit, like apples, eat the skin as well.

For more information, see the Watch Points on page 100.

LIQUIDS

Whether you are dieting or not, your body needs a minimum of 2 litres of liquid a day. Drinking lots of water – from the tap, filtered, mineral or no-calorie flavoured waters, according to your preference – is a good idea, and the remainder may be made up with hot or cold drinks.

Low-carb dieters may wish to avoid caffeine (contained in tea, coffee, hot chocolate, cola, etc.) because it may trigger the production of insulin, and so impair weight loss (see The principles of a low-carb diet, page 5). I suggest that you drink weak black tea or coffee at first (add cream, not milk, if you like it white). Alternatively, choose caffeine-free ones or try herb tea. I would stress, though, that coffee and cocoa contain small amounts of carbohydrates, so if you drink a lot you have to include them in your counting; tea has none. You may also have no-carbohydrate (diet) soft drinks, carbohydrate-free clear soup, pure lemon or lime juice, well diluted with water and artificially sweetened, if necessary. (There is a trace of carbohydrates in them but not as much as in other fruit juices.)

Do not drink milk, sweet pure fruit juices or soft drinks sweetened with sugar.

ALCOHOL

When you are on a low-carbohydrate diet, alcohol doesn't have to be avoided completely but only some types are allowed. Follow these guidelines:

- You may have dry red wine and spirits as they have only a trace of carbohydrates. Remember, though, that your body can derive energy easily from alcohol, so it will burn that before any fat. Ideally, avoid alcohol for the first two weeks when you want to achieve the maximum weight loss.

- Always have no-calorie mixers with spirits.

- Drink plenty of water before and after drinking alcohol. Eat foods high in protein when drinking alcohol so that the body will process them together.

- Dry white, rosé and dry fortified wines have 1–2 g carbohydrates per average glass so should not be included until you reach Phase 3 (see page 177), and are having enough 'healthy' carbohydrates to allow treats.

- Avoid beers, sweet wines, sweet fortified wines and liqueurs as they are high in carbohydrates.

Your Low-carbohydrate Diet

This diet plan is divided into four stages, or phases. The first is very low in carbohydrates to initiate a quick weight loss. The middle phases are designed to help you lose weight whilst still eating a diet that contains all the nutrition your body needs. The last one is a maintenance plan for that time when you've reached your goal and want to remain on a healthy eating regime for life.

The Phases of Your Diet

Full details of each phase, including menus, recipes and lists of permitted foods, are included later in the book.

PHASE 1: QUICK WEIGHT LOSS

Phase 1 is designed to kick-start your diet with an immediate rapid loss of weight. This is done by cutting out most carbohydrates, limiting them to just 20 g per day. On pages 23–27 you will find 14 days of delicious, nutritious menus, with each day's dishes adding up to a total of 20 g. You will notice that, unlike many low-carb diet regimes, this one includes lots of salads and vegetables. It is important that you eat **everything** on the day's menu. So rather than feeling you are restricting your diet, you're being encouraged to eat!

The 14 days' menus are designed to make your diet as simple and enjoyable as possible, and you can simply work your way through them as they are presented, or swap whole days around if you prefer. However, on pages 19–22 you will find a comprehensive list of food items that you are allowed to eat during these first two weeks. If a menu contains something that you dislike, you can substitute a food item with the same carbohydrate content from the list on pages 19-22. So, for example, if you hate cabbage (2 g carbohydrate per serving), you can have runner beans (also 2 g carbohydrate per serving) instead. But you must never just leave something out. It goes without saying you can substitute any meat, fish or poultry for another – you can eat as much as you like of them.

Whatever you choose, you must limit your carbohydrate intake to 20 g per day, and you must eat everything on each day's menu. This regime should be followed for **two weeks only**. Do not be tempted to continue any longer, as the lack of carbohydrates can cause damage to your health.

PHASE 2: GRADUAL WEIGHT LOSS

After two weeks, you progress to the second phase, when you start increasing your daily carbohydrate intake by a small amount each week. You should continue to lose weight gradually, while including more carbohydrate in your diet. It is rather like balancing a delicate set of scales: each person must find the level that suits them. We each burn carbs at a different rate, and this will also vary according to how active we are, so there are no hard-and-fast rules. The guidelines starting on page 99 will help you to find the regime best suited to you. Your weight loss must be gradual if it is to stay off in the long term. If you try to rush it by 'starving' yourself of carbohydrates, you could harm your health and it won't work!

During this phase, the range of foods you can eat is vastly increased. You can make up your meals, choosing ingredients from the lists of individual foods in that section, or you can use the selection of fabulous recipes in the chapter. Either way, you can pick and mix to create your own menus. For each food, I have given the carb content per portion so you can calculate your intake exactly. You can also use the menus from Phase 1, adding extra items from a recommended list as necessary to raise the level of your carbohydrate intake.

Weigh yourself each week (see page 14) during this phase. You should aim to increase your carbohydrates gradually, whilst still steadily continuing to lose weight, until you have nearly reached your target weight. Exactly how long this takes will depend on how much weight you have to lose and how fast your body burns fat. When you have almost reached your target weight, it's time to move on to Phase 3.

PHASE 3: TIME FOR TREATS

By the time you reach this phase, you will have lost most of the weight you want to shed. This phase is designed to help you start to look towards a long-term eating plan by introducing a few treats, such as a small jacket potato, a peach or a slice of bread – the kind of thing that we all like to eat when we are 'eating normally'. This is what the diet is intended to do – it offers you a way to eat those 'normal' foods, whilst still checking that your weight continues to fall, albeit more slowly now.

During Phase 3, you should continue to use the recipes from the first two stages of the diet, maintaining the same carbohydrate intake that you had reached at the end of Phase 2. Now, two or three times a week, you can choose from the list of treats on pages 179-80. Take note of their carbohydrate content and continue to monitor your weight weekly. If you start putting weight on, reduce the number of treats. On the other hand, if you're still losing quickly, you can have an extra treat or two. Alternatively, you can have additional carbohydrates from the lists of those already allowed. Just make a note of what carbohydrates you've eaten, so you can increase or decrease accordingly.

PHASE 4: MAINTAINING THE NEW YOU

Phase 4 isn't really a phase – it is your plan for life. It starts once you have reached your goal, and you are the desired weight or size you want to be. Your diet can now include any fruit and vegetables, and a certain amount of things like bread, potatoes, rice and pasta. However, you should go easy on butter, cream and other fatty foods.

As so often in life, moderation is the key to success here. Yes, you can eat a little of almost anything you like (although I would prefer that you eat whole grain products and give processed foods a miss most of the time). But you must continue to keep an eye on how much carbohydrate you eat, particularly keeping cakes, biscuits and other sugary foods for treats and special occasions.

Starting on page 181, you will find lots of information and tips on how you can eat well and still maintain your weight at your ideal level. There's no need to make special meals for yourself either. Pages 188–204 contain a wonderful selection of delicious recipes that that you can share with family and friends, without worrying about putting on weight. In fact all the recipes in the book make great eating for everybody: simply add a small portion of higher carbohydrate food, such as a small portion of potatoes with a main course or a slice of toast at breakfast.

You will find it very helpful to use a carbohydrate counter to check everything you are eating. *The Hugely Better Carbohydrate Counter* (published by W. Foulsham, 0-572-02958-6) covers almost everything you're likely to eat at home and when dining out. By doing this, you will be able to enjoy your food but know exactly how to keep your weight where you want it.

Starting Your Low-carbohydrate Diet

Before you begin: It is important that you check with your doctor that you are fit and will not suffer any health problems by embarking on this diet. If, for instance, you are already on a low-fat regime, or on a low-cholesterol diet for medical reasons, it may not be suitable for you to go on a low-carbohydrate diet. In particular, if you are diabetic, it is very unlikely that this type of diet would be suitable for you as it would be almost impossible to keep your blood sugar levels low and stable.

IDENTIFY HOW MUCH YOU HAVE TO LOSE

Before starting the diet, you need to establish exactly what your target weight is. You may need to trim only a few pounds – but it may be that you have a lot more to lose.

Overleaf is a chart, based on UK government statistics, which shows you how much you should weigh according to your height. Whether you are at the lower end of the scale or higher up depends on your bone structure. The important thing is that you should be within the limits of your ideal weight.

Weigh yourself first thing in the morning, preferably without clothes. If you weigh yourself with any clothes on, make sure you wear similar garments each time. Look at the scale, then work out how much weight you need to lose. Once you've made that calculation and started on your diet, weigh yourself regularly, but not every day. Once a week is quite enough.

Check Your Weight

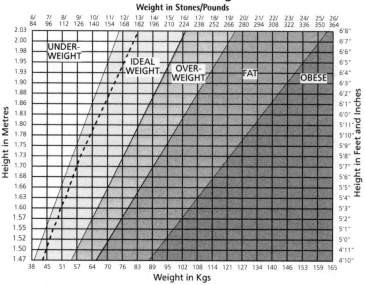

Perhaps you want to drop a couple of dress sizes, in order to get into a new outfit for a special occasion. Record your body measurements, too, before you start your diet. Measure your chest/bust, waist and hips and make a note of the measurements round your upper arm, your thighs, calves and neck. Once you are well into your diet, you will be able to check how much body mass you've lost even if your weight loss slows down considerably. It is interesting to note that lean muscle tissue weighs more than fat. This means that as you continue with your diet, you may find you become smaller in size even if you aren't still actually losing weight.

Notes on the Recipes

- All ingredients are given in imperial, metric and American measures. Follow one set only in a recipe. American terms are given in brackets.

- The ingredients are listed in the order in which they are used in the recipes.

- All spoon measures are level unless otherwise stated: 1 tsp = 5 ml; 1 tbsp = 15 ml.

- Eggs are medium unless otherwise stated.

- Always wash, peel, core and seed, if necessary, fresh produce before use.

- Seasoning and the use of strongly flavoured ingredients such as garlic or chillies are very much a matter of personal taste. Use less than recommended if you prefer. Keep salt to a minimum.

- Always use fresh herbs unless dried are specifically called for. If you wish to substitute dried for fresh, use only half the quantity or less, as they are very pungent. Frozen, chopped varieties have a better colour and flavour than the dried ones if fresh have been called for.

- All can and packet sizes are approximate as they vary from brand to brand.

- All fruit and vegetables are medium-sized unless stated otherwise.

- In some cases I have given a suggested size for pieces of meat, fish and chicken. However, you can have more or less according to your appetite – it won't affect your carbohydrate counts – but don't be greedy!

- Cooking times are approximate and should be used as a guide only. Always check food is piping hot and cooked through before serving.

- Always cook on the shelf just above the centre unless otherwise stated.

- It is not necessary to preheat a fan oven.

- Many of the dishes – especially on the first phase – serve one, as I am assuming you are on the diet alone. All recipes can easily be converted to serve two, four or even more if required.

- Remember, to check the carbohydrate content of everything, from stock cubes to calorie-free drinks … but don't become paranoid. For instance, a stock cube may contain 1.2 g carbohydrate but you'd probably only use the whole cube in a recipe that serves four people, which makes it low in carbohydrate per portion.

- The granular artificial sweetener in the recipes is only a tenth of the weight of ordinary sugar, so never try to weigh it: measure it by volume only (e.g. spoon or cup measures). Also note that when heated too much it can taste very bitter. If you have a sweet tooth and want to add extra to a recipe, do so a very little at a time.

- I have called for butter in the recipes but there is no reason why you shouldn't use margarine if you prefer. Note, however, that low-fat varieties tend to be higher in carbohydrates – so read the labels.

- You may wish to personalise recipes by substituting ingredients. If they contain carbohydrates, make sure you exchange like for like.

- I have used alcohol in some of the recipes. However, it will not affect your diet either because the quantity is too small or because it is cooked, so that it has already evaporated.

- If you are concerned that caffeine may slow down your weight loss, use decaffeinated coffee both in recipes and for drinking.

Phase 1:
Quick Weight Loss

This phase is designed to start your diet off with a rapid, noticeable weight loss. In order to achieve this, you must restrict your carbohydrate intake to just 20 g per day, eating only those foods included in the list on pages 19–22 and in the recommended menus on pages 23–7.

> **This part of the diet is for two weeks only. You should not, under any circumstances, stay on it for longer even if you are thrilled with your rapid weight loss and still have lots to lose.**

Watch points
LIGHT-HEADEDNESS
It is possible that you may feel light-headed early on because of the sudden lack of starch in your diet. If this happens, nibble a small finger of hard cheese. It has only a tiny amount of carbohydrates in it but it will stop that dizzy feeling.

NAUSEA
Some people also feel nauseous. This is because of the change in your protein and fat intake. I suggest sipping sparkling water, either plain or flavoured with pure lemon or lime juice. If you have a sweet tooth, an artificially sweetened flavoured seltzer is a good idea or 'diet' ginger ale. Another good remedy is to sip mint tea.

UPSET TUMMY
It is quite common for people to get diarrhoea when they first embark on a low-carbohydrate diet. It happens particularly if the person is not used to eating lots of raw salad stuffs. If you have wind as well, try lightly cooking vegetables and dressing them with oil and vinegar instead of having raw salads. It is important to chew all raw vegetables thoroughly because otherwise they are difficult to digest.

Another cause can be the added fat in your diet. If you were on a low-fat regime before, the added oils, butter and cream could be enough to cause your upset tummy. Provided you are not in pain, the problem should right itself.

If you are using a lot of artificial sweeteners, it may be these causing the problem, either because they contain sorbitol, which has a laxative effect, or because they contain maltodextrin as a bulky filler to make it more like ordinary sugar. This, too, can cause diarrhoea in some people.

If you have serious bloating, flatulence and cramp-like pains, you may have a food intolerance or irritable bowel syndrome. Seek medical advice before continuing with the diet.

KETOSIS

You don't have to suffer ketosis if you don't want to. If the symptoms start, (the metallic taste in the mouth and bad breath), eat a 'rescue food': a small raw carrot or half a red (bell) pepper. You can do this every day if necessary to prevent the problem (see page 6 for more about ketosis).

CRAVINGS AND HUNGER PANGS

You should find your craving for sweet foods diminishes. However, I have included desserts on this regime because most people feel happier if they have them and are more likely to stick to the diet if they aren't deprived of them. If you don't fancy something sweet, you can always have cheese with some extra salad vegetables to add up to the number of carbohydrates the dessert provided (see pages 20–22 for the carbohydrate values of different permitted foods).

Theoretically, you shouldn't feel hungry between meals on this diet but if you do feel desperately peckish, nibble a no-carbohydrate snack, such as a small finger of hard cheese, a slice of lean ham or a chicken drumstick. Alternatively, try making a hot drink of Bovril or Marmite. Ideally, however, you should stick to eating just the meals and drinking plenty of water in between. Sipping sparkling mineral water or a no-calorie/no-carbohydrate sparkling flavoured drink will also help to stave off hunger pangs. Do eat enough at every meal to fill you up and, if necessary, have larger portions of meat, fish, poultry or cheese. But don't do this just because you can. Over-eating will be counter-productive as any food you eat over and above what your body needs will simply slow down your weight loss. Remember the old saying: 'Enough is as good as a feast!'

Foods you are allowed

You do not have to stick slavishly to the menus if you don't want to. However, you must not exceed your daily allowance of 20 g carbohydrates. The following list tells you which foods you can – or can't – eat.

EAT IN UNLIMITED QUANTITIES

Some foods do not contain any carbohydrates, so you can eat as much as you like. Where these are included in my menus, you can have larger or smaller portions, depending on your appetite.

Pure meat and poultry

You can eat beef, pork, lamb, veal, bacon, gammon, ham, rabbit, venison, chicken, turkey, duck, goose, pheasant, quail, grouse and other game. Note that some offal, such as liver, is extremely nutritious but does contain a small amount of carbohydrate, so I have limited it at this stage.

Pure fish and shellfish

You are permitted all white fish, such as cod, haddock and sole; oily fish, such as tuna, salmon, sardines and mackerel; and seafood, such as prawns (shrimp), crab (not dressed crab, however, as it contains breadcrumbs), lobster, oysters, mussels, clams and squid.

All hard and fresh cheeses

You can eat everything from Cheddar and Edam to Stilton and Dolcelatte, Mozzarella and Camembert, plus goats' and sheep's cheeses. Note that some cheeses have small amounts of carbohydrate in them, so where necessary I have included these in the calculations. Whey cheeses, such as ricotta, should be avoided during the first two weeks.

Olive, seed and vegetable oils

Butter, fresh creams and crème fraîche

Note that single (light) and soured (dairy sour) cream have 1 g carbohydrate per 15 ml/tablespoon, so, when used in the diet, are included in the carbohydrate count. Don't have too much of these, however, especially on the first quick-loss phase, when each gram of carbohydrate counts. There is no reason why you shouldn't eat margarine instead of butter. The only reason some low-carbohydrate diets ban it is because the fat is processed and so it contains trans fatty acids, which aren't good for you. However, too much animal fat isn't either, so if you prefer to use a sunflower margarine, for instance, instead of butter, do so. With all margarines and creams, beware of the low-fat ones as they tend to have higher carbohydrates. Always check the labels.

Eggs

These may be cooked any way.

EAT IN RESTRICTED QUANTITIES

Some foods you can eat only in specified quantities that keep within the carbohydrate allowance.

Vegetables

The carbohydrate counts below are based on an average-sized portion of 100 g/4 oz/3 heaped tbsp unless stated otherwise. You can only eat those vegetables that have a very low carbohydrate content, i.e. less than 10 g per portion. If you eat any of the vegetables raw, add on 1 g per serving.

Item	Carb content per portion
Artichoke hearts – 1 heart	1 g
Asparagus	2 g
Aubergine (eggplant) – ½ medium	3 g
Bamboo shoots	trace
Beansprouts – a good handful	1 g
Broccoli	2 g
Brussels sprouts	3 g
Cabbage, all types	2 g

Item	Carb content per portion
Carrots *	5 g
Cauliflower	2 g
Celeriac (celery root)	2 g
Courgettes (zucchini)	3 g
French (green) beans	5 g
Kale	1 g
Kohlrabi	5 g
Leeks	3 g
Mangetout (snow peas)	2 g
Marrow (squash)	2 g
Mushrooms, all types	trace
Okra	3 g
Onions – 1 medium	7 g
Pak choi	2 g
Palm hearts – 1 piece	2 g
Pumpkin	2 g
Rhubarb	1 g
Runner beans	2 g
Spinach	1 g
Spring (collard) greens	2 g
Swede (rutabaga)	2 g
Swiss chard	4 g
Turnip	2 g
Water chestnuts	3 g

* Some low-carbohydrate diets say you shouldn't have carrots at this stage because they contain sugars. But when cooked they contain only 5 g carbohydrate (8 g in a large raw one) and are a good source of fibre, so I have included them.

Fruit
Only a few fruits are permitted at this stage.

Item	Carb content per item
Avocado – 1 medium	3 g
Olives	trace
Tomato – 1 medium	2 g

Salad stuffs

If you cook any of these, such as celery, take off 1 g per serving.

Item	Carb content per portion
Celery	1 g
Chicory (Belgian endive) – 1 medium	2 g
Cucumber – 5 slices	1 g
Fennel – ½ head	2 g
Fresh herbs	trace
Lettuce, all types – a good handful	1 g
(Bell) peppers – 1 medium	green, 4 g
	yellow/orange, 7 g
	red, 10 g
Radishes – each	trace
Rocket – a good handful	trace
Sorrel – a good handful	trace
Watercress – a good handful	trace

Spices

You can eat all types provided there is no starchy filler or sugar in the mix.

DO NOT EAT

You may not eat any of the following:

- Processed meat, poultry and fish products that contain carbohydrates, e.g. sausages, fish fingers, southern fried chicken – check the labels

- Milk and yoghurt

- Fruits, apart from the three listed on page 21

- Starchy foods, such as bread, potatoes, pasta, rice or other grains

- Sugar of any kind and foods containing any type of sugar

Phase 1 Meal Planner

DAY 1

Breakfast Baked Eggs in Tomatoes with Cheese (see page 28)

              Coffee or tea (black or with a dash of cream)

Lunch   Caesar Salad with Anchovies and Crispy Bacon
(see page 44)

              Strawberry sugar-free jelly

Dinner   Sirloin Steak with Mushrooms in Garlic Butter
(see page 59)

              Moreish and Golden Celeriac Chips (see page 58)

              Venetian Coffee Cream Cheese (see page 80)

DAY 2

Breakfast Grilled Bacon with Buttery Pan-stewed Flat Mushrooms
(see page 29)

              Coffee or tea (black or with a dash of cream)

Lunch   Tomato Soup with Fresh Basil (see page 42)

              Mixed Cheese Platter with Fennel (see page 87)

Dinner   Greek Aubergine Moussaka (see page 60)

              Lamb's Tongue Lettuce and Radish Salad (see page 61)

              Rhubarb with Creamy Custard Sauce (see page 82)

DAY 3

Breakfast Grilled Kipper with Creamy Scrambled Eggs (see page 30)

              Coffee or tea (black or with a dash of cream)

Lunch   Seviche with Avocado, Pepper and Chilli (see page 43)

              Refreshing Summer Fruit Frostie (see page 81)

Dinner   Grilled Cheese-topped Gammon with Courgettes
(see page 62)

              Rum and Chocolate Mousse (see page 84)

Day 4

Breakfast Devilled Lambs' Kidneys with Mushrooms (see page 32)

Coffee or Tea (black or with a dash of cream)

Lunch Tomato, Artichoke, Rocket and Mozzarella Salad (see page 46)

Grilled Avocado Slices with Crème Fraîche (see page 83)

Dinner Pan-roasted Chicken with Mushrooms and Turnips (see page 64)

A green salad (see page 65)

Fresh Lemon and Lime Sorbet (see page 86)

Day 5

Breakfast Home-made Sausages with Tomatoes (see page 31)

Coffee or tea (black or with a dash of cream)

Lunch Cauliflower in Baked Cheese Sauce (see page 47)

Orange sugar-free jelly

Dinner Warm Salmon Salad with Asparagus (see page 63)

Light and Creamy Mocha Whip (see page 85)

Day 6

Breakfast Victorian-style Mumbled Eggs with Cream Cheese (see page 34)

Coffee or tea (black or with a dash of cream)

Lunch Beef Consommé with Chicken (see page 45)

Chunky Tuna Mayonnaise Salad with Paprika (see page 48)

Emmental with Radishes and Black Pepper (see page 87)

Dinner Lamb Shank with Rosemary Jus (see page 66)

Creamy Celeriac and Carrot Mash (see page 67)

Peppery Wild Rocket Salad (see page 67)

Smooth Baked Vanilla Cream (see page 88)

Day 7

Breakfast Traditional Bacon and Eggs in One Pan (see page 33)

Coffee or tea (black or with a dash of cream)

Lunch Grilled Goats' Cheese Salad with Walnut Oil Dressing (see page 49)

St Clements Jelly with Crème Fraîche (see page 89)

Dinner Roast Pork with Swede and Roasted Onions (see page 68)

Mangetout

Creamy Chocolate Custard Dessert (see page 90)

Day 8

Breakfast Baked Eggs with Ham and Cream (see page 36)

Coffee or tea (black or with a dash of cream)

Lunch Greek Village Salad with Feta, Olives and Oregano (see page 50)

Chilled Lime Crème (see page 89)

Dinner Grilled Mackerel with Mustard Rub (see page 74)

Carrots

Runner beans

Mediterranean-style Coffee Granita (see page 91)

Day 9

Breakfast Giant Stuffed Mushrooms with Ham and Cheese (see page 35)

Coffee or tea (black or with a dash of cream)

Lunch Curried Egg Mayonnaise with Watercress (see page 51)

Cheese and Sun-dried Tomato-stuffed Celery (see page 45)

Dinner Liver, Bacon and Savoy with Onion Gravy (see page 70)

Crushed Swede with Butter and Cream (see page 71)

Quick and Easy Lemon Snow (see page 93)

Day 10

Breakfast Poached Eggs with Spinach and Creamed Mushrooms (see page 38)

Coffee or tea (black or with a dash of cream)

Lunch Sliced Aubergine and Mozzarella Grill (see page 52)

Fresh Lemon and Lime Sorbet (see page 86)

Dinner Chicken and Bamboo Shoots with Pak Choi (see page 69)

Blue-cheese-stuffed Cucumber (see page 94)

Day 11

Breakfast Grilled Halloumi Cheese with Bacon (see page 37)

Coffee or tea (black or with a dash of cream)

Lunch Button Mushroom and Chive Omelette (see page 53)

Rich and Creamy Strawberry Mousse Layer (see page 95)

Dinner Grilled Tuna with Peppers and Olives (see page 72)

Garlic-sautéed Courgettes (see page 71)

Melted Camembert with Blackcurrant and Celery (see page 96)

Day 12

Breakfast Pan-scrambled Eggs with Ham (see page 40)

Coffee or tea (black or with a dash of cream)

Lunch Avocado with Prawns in Thousand Island Dressing (see page 54)

Raspberry sugar-free jelly

Dinner Peppered Pork Chop with Sautéed Caraway Cabbage (see page 76)

Okra Provençale with Spring Onions and Garlic (see page 77)

Fresh Lemon and Lime Sorbet (see page 86)

Day 13

Breakfast Golden Soufflé Omelette with Herbs (see page 39)

Coffee or tea (black or with a dash of cream)

Lunch Chilled Cream of Cucumber Soup with Dill (see page 55)

Ham, Cream Cheese and Asparagus Rolls (see page 57)

Dinner Beef Stroganoff with Mushrooms and Brandy
(see page 78)

Broccoli and Cauliflower Sauté (see page 79)

Rhubarb Fool with Fresh Ginger (see page 97)

Day 14

Breakfast Bacon with Celeriac and Onion Hash Browns (see page 41)

Coffee or tea (black or with a dash of cream)

Lunch Grilled Chicken Legs in Lemon and Garlic Marinade
(see page 56)

Lettuce and Cucumber Rolls with Cheddar (see page 57)

Blackcurrant Fluff (see page 96)

Dinner Warm Smoked Haddock and Quails' Egg Salad
(see page 73)

Almond-flavoured Jelly Cream (see page 98)

Breakfast Recipes

All these recipes are specifically designed for Phase 1, but you can obviously continue to use them throughout the diet. As your carbohydrate allowance increases in later phases, you can top it up from other sources, as explained later in the book.

Baked eggs in tomatoes with cheese

Large juicy tomatoes make perfect nests for eggs, topped with golden, melted cheese. They are ideal for a not-too-heavy breakfast or even for a lunch dish.

2 beefsteak tomatoes

A little olive oil

2 large eggs

Freshly ground black pepper

25 g/1 oz/¼ cup grated Cheddar cheese

1 Preheat the oven to 180°C/350°F/ gas 4/fan oven 160°C. Cut a slice off the rounded end of the tomatoes and scoop out the seeds.

2 Stand the shells in a lightly oiled individual dish and brush inside with olive oil.

3 Break an egg into each tomato, season with pepper, then top with the cheese.

4 Bake in the oven for 12–15 minutes for soft-cooked eggs, 20 minutes if you like the yolks hard.

Serves 1
Carbohydrates: 8 g

Grilled bacon with buttery flat mushrooms

Large flat mushrooms have a wonderful earthy flavour, especially when stewed with butter and lots of black pepper. They marry perfectly with bacon for a delicious start to the day.

1 Peel the mushrooms.

2 Melt the butter in a large frying pan (skillet). Add the mushrooms, gill-sides up, and season with salt and pepper. Fry (sauté) for 2–3 minutes, then loosen them with a fish slice if they have stuck to the pan.

3 Add the water, cover the pan with a lid or foil, turn down the heat and stew for 5 minutes.

4 Meanwhile, grill (broil) the bacon for 3–4 minutes, turning once, until golden and sizzling.

5 Transfer the mushrooms and any remaining juices to a warm plate, add the bacon, then serve.

4 large flat mushrooms

A knob of butter

Salt and freshly ground black pepper

45 ml/3 tbsp water

2 rashers (slices) of back bacon, rinded

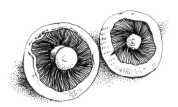

Serves 1

Carbohydrates: Trace

Grilled kipper with creamy scrambled eggs

Kippers make a perfect accompaniment to soft, lightly cooked, scrambled eggs. If you don't like kippers, you can substitute smoked salmon or grilled bacon, or make extra scrambled eggs.

1 kipper, on the bone or filleted

15 g/½ oz/1 tbsp butter

2 eggs

30 ml/2 tbsp double (heavy) cream

Salt and freshly ground black pepper

1 Put the kipper skin-side up on foil on the grill (broiler) rack. Grill (broil) for 2 minutes. Turn the fish over and dot with half the butter. Grill for a further 2–3 minutes until cooked through and sizzling.

2 Meanwhile, melt the remaining butter in a small saucepan. Whisk in the eggs, cream and a little salt and pepper. Cook over a gentle heat, stirring all the time, until scrambled but still creamy.

3 Transfer the fish and eggs to a warm plate and serve.

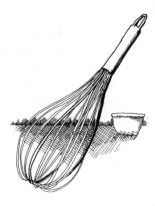

Serves 1

Carbohydrates: Trace

Home-made sausages with tomatoes

It's not worth making a smaller number of sausages. If eating alone, freeze the rest. You may eat more or fewer as they contain no carbs, but eat only two tomatoes.

1 Cut the rind off the belly pork slices and cut out any bones. Cut into chunks.

2 Pick over the bacon, discarding any bones, gristle or rind. Cut into smaller pieces, if necessary.

3 Drop the pork and bacon a piece at a time into a food processor with the machine running until finely chopped, or pass through a mincer (grinder).

4 Season with the herbs and lots of pepper.

5 Draw the mixture together into a ball. Remove any white stringy bits of gristly pork fat that haven't chopped.

6 Shape the mixture into small sausages or balls.

7 Place the sausages and tomato halves on foil on a grill (broiler) rack. Drizzle the tomatoes with a little olive oil. Grill (broil) for about 5–6 minutes, turning the sausages occasionally until golden and cooked through. Turn the tomatoes once. Alternatively, fry (sauté) the sausages and tomatoes in in a little olive oil for a similar amount of time.

8 Serve hot.

450 g/1 lb belly pork slices

225 g/8 oz bacon pieces

5 ml/1 tsp dried mixed herbs

Freshly ground black pepper

8 tomatoes, halved

Olive oil

Serves 4

Carbohydrates: 4 g per serving

Devilled lambs' kidneys with mushrooms

A taste of the old days! Succulent kidneys spiked with spices and bathed in a rich sauce – a substantial breakfast to enjoy at your leisure and set you up for the day.

2 lambs' kidneys

25 g/1 oz/2 tbsp butter

1.5 ml/¼ tsp chilli powder

1.5 ml/¼ tsp made English mustard

1.5 ml/¼ tsp paprika

15 ml/1 tbsp tomato purée (paste)

Salt and freshly ground black pepper

A pinch of artificial sweetener

6 button mushrooms, halved or quartered

1 Remove any skin from the kidneys and cut out the central cores with scissors. Cut into bite-sized pieces.

2 Melt the butter in a frying pan (skillet). Add the kidneys and fry (sauté), stirring, for 3 minutes until brown but still soft.

3 Add the chilli, mustard, paprika and tomato purée and stir until thoroughly blended. Season to taste with salt, pepper and sweetener. Simmer for 1–2 minutes, stirring.

4 Spoon into a warm, shallow bowl and serve with the raw mushrooms to mop up the juices.

Serves 1
Carbohydrates: 2 g

Traditional bacon and eggs in one pan

Most people love a fry-up - that wonderful aroma, filling the kitchen. I prefer to grill the bacon and poach the eggs - but the choice is yours. Cook more if you like.

1 Heat the oil in a frying pan (skillet). Add the bacon and fry (sauté) for 2 minutes until golden underneath.

2 Turn the bacon over and push to one side of the pan. Break in the eggs and season well with pepper. Fry, spooning the oil over the yolks, until cooked to your liking.

3 Transfer the bacon and eggs to a warm plate and serve.

30 ml/2 tbsp sunflower oil

2 rashers (slices) of bacon, rinded

2 eggs

Freshly ground black pepper

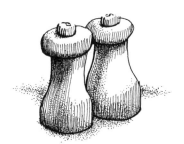

Serves 1

Carbohydrates: 0 g

Victorian-style mumbled eggs with cream cheese

An old-fashioned recipe created when people took time over their breakfasts, so make sure you get up early, so that you can sit down and really relish the subtle flavours.

1 tomato, sliced

30 ml/2 tbsp whipping cream

25 g/1 oz/2 tbsp cream cheese

2 eggs

2.5 ml/½ tsp made English mustard

Salt and freshly ground black pepper

1 Arrange the tomato slices in a circle on a plate. Place in a very low oven to warm.

2 Put the cream and cheese in a saucepan and heat gently, stirring until smooth.

3 Remove from the heat and whisk in the eggs, mustard and a little salt and pepper.

4 Return to the heat and cook gently, stirring, until just set but still creamy.

5 Spoon into the centre of the tomato ring and serve.

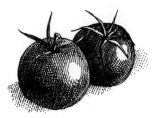

Serves 1
Carbohydrates: 2 g

Giant stuffed mushrooms with ham and cheese

Enormous mushrooms, cradling slices of lean, cured ham, lifted with just a dash of Worcestershire sauce and smothered in mild Edam cheese.

1 Peel the mushrooms and trim off the stalks. Brush all over with the oil and sprinkle with lots of pepper.

2 Place gill-sides down on foil on the grill (broiler) rack. Cook under a preheated grill for 3 minutes until turning golden.

3 Turn the mushrooms over. Put a slice of ham in each mushroom, folding it to fit. Sprinkle each with a few drops of Worcestershire sauce, then top with the cheese. Grill (broil) for a further 3 minutes until the cheese melts and bubbles.

4 Slide on to a warm plate and pour any juices over.

2 very large cup mushrooms

15 ml/1 tbsp olive oil

Freshly ground black pepper

2 slices of ham

A few drops of Worcestershire sauce

25 g/1 oz/¼ cup grated Edam cheese

Serves 1
Carbohydrates: 1 g

Baked eggs with ham and cream

A civilised breakfast of eggs, nestling on pieces of succulent ham, bathed in cream to keep them deliciously soft, this makes a wonderful start to the day.

A little olive oil, for greasing

2 slices of lean cooked ham, diced

2 eggs

Salt and pepper

30 ml/2 tbsp double (heavy) cream

1 Grease two ramekin dishes (custard cups) with a little olive oil.

2 Put the diced ham in the bases, then break an egg into each dish.

3 Season with salt and pepper, then add the cream. Place in a roasting tin (pan) containing enough boiling water to come halfway up the sides of the dishes.

4 Bake in a preheated oven at 180°C/ 350°F/gas 4/fan oven 160°C for 10–15 minutes until cooked to your liking.

Serves 1

Carbohydrates: Trace

Grilled Halloumi cheese with bacon

A touch of the Mediterranean here - slices of firm, slightly salty Halloumi cheese, drizzled with olive oil, spiked with lemon and herbs and grilled until golden with smoked bacon.

1 Put the cheese on foil on a grill (broiler) rack and drizzle with the oil. Add a squeeze of lemon, then sprinkle with the herbs and lots of pepper. Lay the bacon alongside.

2 Cook under a preheated grill for 3–4 minutes until the cheese and bacon are lightly golden.

3 Serve hot.

3 slices of Halloumi cheese, about 5 mm/¼ in thick

15 ml/1 tbsp olive oil

A squeeze of lemon juice

3 pinches of dried oregano

Freshly ground black pepper

2 rashers (slices) of smoked back bacon, rinded

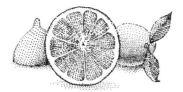

Serves 1
Carbohydrates: 1 g

Poached eggs with spinach and creamed mushrooms

A gourmet breakfast of softly poached eggs set on lightly cooked, tender young spinach coated in a creamy mushroom sauce - a wonderful combination of textures and flavours.

A small knob of butter

50 g/2 oz button mushrooms, thinly sliced

30 ml/2 tbsp crème fraîche

A good pinch of onion salt

Freshly ground black pepper

100 g/4 oz fresh young spinach

2 eggs

2 tsp lemon juice or vinegar

1 Melt the butter in a saucepan. Add the mushrooms and cook, stirring, for 2 minutes. Stir in the crème fraîche and season with the onion salt and lots of pepper.

2 Wash the spinach thoroughly and place in a saucepan with no extra water. Cover and cook over a gentle heat, stirring once or twice, for 3 minutes until just softened but not mushy. Drain thoroughly.

3 Meanwhile, poach the eggs in simmering water, with the lemon juice or vinegar added, for 3–4 minutes until cooked to your liking. (You can use an egg poacher if you prefer.)

4 Reheat the mushrooms. Put the spinach on a warm plate. Top with the eggs and spoon the creamed mushrooms over.

Serves 1

Carbohydrates: 1 g

Golden soufflé omelette with herbs

Light and delicious, this plain, fluffy soufflé omelette is heightened with fragrant herbs and makes a perfect, not-too-heavy start to the day.

1 Beat the egg yolks and water together with a little salt and pepper. Stir in the fresh and dried herbs.

2 Whisk the egg whites until stiff and fold into the yolk mixture with a metal spoon.

3 Melt the butter in an omelette pan. When hot, spoon in the soufflé mixture and spread out evenly. Cook gently for about 3–4 minutes until golden underneath and partially set. Meanwhile, preheat the grill (broiler).

4 Put the omelette in its pan under the grill and cook until puffy and golden brown. Serve immediately.

2 eggs, separated

10 ml/2 tsp water

Salt and freshly ground black pepper

5 ml/1 tsp chopped fresh parsley

A good pinch of dried mixed herbs

15 g/½ oz/1 tbsp butter

Serves 1

Carbohydrates: 0 g

Pan-scrambled eggs with ham

This dish is equally delicious made with a handful of smoked-salmon trimmings instead of ham – either way it makes a really sumptuous breakfast.

2 eggs

30 ml/2 tbsp water

Salt and freshly ground black pepper

A knob of butter

10 ml/2 tsp chopped fresh parsley

2 slices of ham, cut into thin shreds

1 Beat the eggs with the water, a pinch of salt and a good grinding of pepper.

2 Melt the butter in a frying pan (skillet). Add the eggs and sprinkle the parsley over. Cook over a fairly gentle heat, stirring occasionally, until they just begin to scramble.

3 Scatter the ham all over the surface and continue to cook, stirring all the time, until the eggs are scrambled.

4 Tip on to a warm plate and serve.

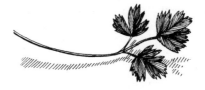

Serves 1

Carbohydrates: 0 g

Bacon with celeriac and onion hash browns

Made with elegant celeriac, these mouth-watering morsels are delicious hot or cold. It's worth cooking a whole celeriac. You can keep it in the fridge for a few days, or freeze it.

1 Boil the celeriac in lightly salted water for about 10 minutes until soft. Drain and tip into a bowl. Mash well.

2 Meanwhile, fry (sauté) the bacon in a frying pan (skillet) until golden, turning once. Remove from the pan and keep warm.

3 Add the oil to the pan and heat. Add the onion and fry for 2 minutes, stirring.

4 Remove from the pan with a draining spoon and add to the celeriac. Mix together well, season with salt and pepper, then mix with the beaten egg.

5 Add the butter to the oil in the frying pan. Heat until bubbling, then add spoonfuls of the celeriac mixture and fry for 2 minutes until golden underneath. Turn the hash browns over and fry the other sides until golden.

6 Drain on kitchen paper (paper towels), then serve with the bacon.

¼ celeriac (celery root), cut into small chunks

2 rashers (slices) of back bacon, rinded

15 ml/1 tbsp sunflower or olive oil

1 small onion, chopped

Salt and freshly ground black pepper

1 egg, beaten

A knob of butter

Serves 1

Carbohydrates: 11 g

Lunch Recipes

Many of these are suitable to take to work for a packed lunch, others are better reserved for eating at home. You'll find all the desserts and other 'afters' at the end of the recipe section.

Tomato soup with fresh basil

A fresh, fragrant soup that's really simple to prepare. It's not worth making soup for one. Serve it to others too or freeze in separate portions for other meals.

15 ml/1 tbsp olive oil

1 onion, finely chopped

500 ml/17 fl oz/ 2¼ cups passata (sieved tomatoes)

250 ml/8 fl oz/1 cup vegetable or chicken stock, made with ½ stock cube

A good pinch of artificial sweetener

Salt and freshly ground black pepper

15 ml/1 tbsp chopped fresh basil, plus a few leaves for garnishing

1 Heat the oil in a saucepan. Add the onion and fry (sauté), stirring over a gentle heat, for 3 minutes until softened but not browned.

2 Add the passata and stock. Bring to the boil, reduce the heat, part-cover and simmer gently for 15 minutes.

3 Season to taste with the sweetener, salt and pepper and stir in the chopped basil.

4 Purée, if liked, in a blender or food processor, then return to the pan. Reheat the soup until piping hot.

5 Serve garnished with a few whole basil leaves.

Serves 4
Carbohydrates: 7 g

Seviche with avocado, pepper and chilli

Chunks of the freshest fish, mixed with pepper, tomato, avocado and onion, spiked with chilli and marinated in fresh citrus and olive oil, served on a bed of endive, garnished with cucumber.

1 Cut the fish into bite-size pieces and put in a bowl, add the lime or lemon juice and toss gently. Chill for at least 3 hours, turning occasionally. It will turn completely white, as if it has been cooked.

2 Add all the remaining ingredients except the endive and cucumber and toss gently. Chill, if possible, for a further hour to allow the flavours to develop.

3 Pile the mixture on to the curly endive and garnish with the cucumber slices.

175 g/6 oz thick white fish, skinned

2 tsp lime or lemon juice

1 tomato, skinned, seeded and diced

½ small green (bell) pepper, diced

½ small green chilli, seeded and chopped

1 spring onion (scallion), chopped

5 ml/1 tsp olive oil

5 ml/1 tsp chopped fresh parsley

2.5 ml/½ tsp white wine vinegar

1 ripe avocado, sliced

Salt and freshly ground black pepper

A good handful of curly endive (frisée lettuce)

5 slices of cucumber

Serves 1
Carbohydrates: 10 g

Caesar salad with anchovies and crispy bacon

Crisp lettuce and crunchy bacon tossed in a garlic and anchovy dressing, then topped with fresh Parmesan. Leftover anchovies can be stored in the fridge for several days or frozen for later use.

½ x 50 g/2 oz/small can of anchovies

2 rashers (slices) of streaky bacon, rinded and diced

¼ small cos (romaine) lettuce, cut into chunky pieces

1 egg

½ small garlic clove, crushed

45 ml/3 tbsp sunflower oil

15 ml/1 tbsp white wine vinegar

2.5 ml/½ tsp Dijon mustard

2.5 ml/½ tsp artificial sweetener

Salt and freshly ground black pepper

25 g/1 oz freshly shaved Parmesan cheese

Serves 1
Carbohydrates: 2 g

1 Put the anchovies in a small bowl. Cover with cold water and leave to soak while preparing the rest of the salad.

2 Dry-fry the bacon in a frying pan (skillet) until crisp and golden. Drain on kitchen paper (paper towels).

3 Put the lettuce in a bowl and sprinkle with the bacon.

4 Put the egg in a pan of cold water. Bring to the boil and boil for just 1½ minutes – no longer – then plunge the egg immediately into cold water.

5 Drain the anchovies and chop one of them. Put it in a bowl with the garlic and work together with a wire whisk.

6 Break the egg into the bowl. Whisk it into the anchovy mixture, then whisk in the oil a little at a time. Finally, add the vinegar, mustard, artificial sweetener and salt and pepper to taste.

7 Cut the remaining anchovies into two or three pieces and add to the lettuce. Pour over the dressing and toss. Scatter the Parmesan shavings over and serve.

Cheese and sun-dried tomato-stuffed celery

A sensational nibble! The sun-dried tomatoes add flavour and piquancy to this popular savoury with its great combination of soft and crisp textures.

1 Mash the cheese with the tomato, adding pepper to taste.
2 Spread along the celery, then cut into short lengths.

25 g/1 oz/generous 1 tbsp cream cheese

1 piece of sun-dried tomato in oil, drained and finely chopped

Freshly ground black pepper

1 large celery stick

Serves 1
Carbohydrates: 2 g

Beef consommé with chicken

If eating alone, make up half and freeze the rest. Try adding diced ham or cooked peeled prawns instead of the chicken. All will boost the taste and add protein with no extra carbs.

1 Make up the consommé as directed on the can. Add the chicken and heat through.
2 Ladle into two warm soup bowls and serve.

1 x 295 g/10¾ oz/ medium can of beef consommé

A handful of diced cooked chicken

Serves 2
Carbohydrates: 1 g per serving

Tomato, artichoke, rocket and Mozzarella salad

A Mediterranean extravaganza of colour, flavour and texture - this makes the perfect lunch dish. You could use a whole sliced avocado instead of the artichokes, and add an extra tomato.

A good handful of rocket

2 cherry tomatoes, quartered

4 canned artichoke hearts, drained and quartered

1 x 100 g/4 oz/small fresh Mozzarella cheese, drained and diced

6 fresh basil leaves, torn

6 black olives

15 ml/1 tbsp olive oil

5 ml/1 tsp balsamic vinegar

Freshly ground black pepper

1 Pile the rocket on a plate.

2 Scatter the tomatoes, artichoke hearts, cheese, basil and olives over the top.

3 Trickle the oil, then the vinegar over the salad and add a good grinding of pepper.

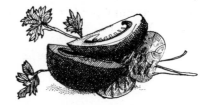

Serves 1
Carbohydrates: 11 g

Cauliflower in baked cheese sauce

This delicious alternative to cauliflower in the traditionally carb-laden cheese sauce makes a light, nutritious and elegant lunch with plenty of flavour.

1 Cook the cauliflower in boiling, lightly salted water for about 5 minutes or until just tender. Drain thoroughly and tip into an ovenproof dish.

2 Whisk the egg, then whisk the crème fraîche and mustard into it. Stir in half the cheese and season with a very little salt and lots of pepper.

3 Spoon this mixture over the cauliflower and sprinkle with the remaining grated cheese.

4 Bake in a preheated oven at 190°C/ 375°F/gas 5/fan oven 170°C for about 35 minutes until golden brown and the sauce is set.

½ small cauliflower, cut into 8 florets

1 egg

45 ml/3 tbsp crème fraîche

30 ml/2 tbsp water

1.5 ml/¼ tsp made English mustard

25 g/1 oz/¼ cup grated Cheddar cheese

Salt and freshly ground black pepper

Serves 1
Carbohydrates: 6 g

Chunky tuna mayonnaise salad with paprika

This is a classic dish of tuna blended with rich, creamy mayonnaise and served on a bed of fresh, green salad to create a complete and appetising dish. Tuna has no carbohydrates.

A good handful of mixed salad leaves

2.5 cm/1 in piece of cucumber, diced

1 tomato, finely diced

1 spring onion (scallion), chopped

½ small green (bell) pepper, cut into thin rings

1 x 85 g/3½ oz/small can of tuna in oil, drained

30 ml/2 tbsp mayonnaise

Freshly ground black pepper

Paprika, for dusting

1 Pile the leaves on a plate and scatter the cucumber, tomato, spring onion and pepper over.

2 Tip the tuna into a bowl and break up into chunks. Fold in the mayonnaise and lots of pepper. Mix together but do take care not to break up the chunks of tuna.

3 Spoon the tuna mayonnaise on to the salad and dust with paprika.

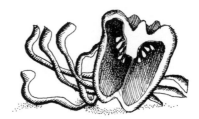

Serves 1
Carbohydrates: 5 g

Grilled goats' cheese salad with walnut oil dressing

Goats' cheese is ideal for grilling as it holds its shape while becoming deliciously soft. Served on a tender green salad, the walnut oil dressing complements it perfectly.

1 Pile the spinach or lettuce on to a plate. Scatter the cucumber, tomato and celery over.

2 Whisk the walnut oil with the vinegar and a good grinding of pepper. Trickle over the salad.

3 Put the cheese on a piece of foil on the grill (broiler) rack. Cook under a preheated grill for 2–3 minutes until lightly golden on top but still holding its shape.

4 Transfer to the bed of salad and serve.

A good handful of baby spinach or lettuce leaves

5 slices of cucumber

1 tomato, sliced

1 celery stick, sliced

15 ml/1 tbsp walnut oil

5 ml/1 tsp balsamic vinegar

Freshly ground black pepper

1 x 70 g/2¾ oz individual round of goats' cheese

Serves 1
Carbohydrates: 6 g

Greek village salad with feta, olives and oregano

Another classic from the Mediterranean - fresh salad mingled with the contrasting colours and flavours of black olives and white feta cheese, dressed with an oil, vinegar and herb dressing.

A good handful of shredded white cabbage

A good handful of shredded iceberg lettuce

1 tomato, cut into wedges

2.5 cm/1 in piece of cucumber, diced

1 thin slice of onion, separated into rings

6 black olives

40 g/1½ oz/¼ cup crumbled feta cheese

15 ml/1 tbsp olive oil

5 ml/1 tsp red wine vinegar

Freshly ground black pepper

1.5 ml/¼ tsp dried oregano

1 Put the shredded cabbage on a plate with the lettuce on top.

2 Scatter the tomato, cucumber, onion and olives over, then top with the crumbled cheese.

3 Trickle the oil and vinegar over and season well with pepper. Finally, sprinkle with the oregano.

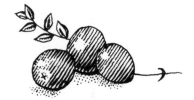

Serves 1

Carbohydrates: 8 g

Curried egg mayonnaise with watercress

A tasty favourite that has stood the test of time: hard-boiled eggs in a spicy mayonnaise on a bed of lettuce and watercress. Halve the quantity of eggs and dressing for a small appetite.

1 Put the eggs in a pan of cold water, bring to the boil and boil for 7 minutes. Drain, cover with cold water and leave until cold. Shell and halve the eggs.

2 Mix the lettuce and watercress together and pile on a plate. Arrange the eggs over.

3 Blend the curry powder with the mayonnaise, lemon juice and sweetener to taste. Spoon over the eggs and dust with a little dried parsley.

2 eggs

A good handful of torn lettuce

A good handful of trimmed watercress

1.5 ml/¼ tsp curry powder

30 ml/2 tbsp mayonnaise

2.5 ml/½ tsp lemon juice

A pinch of artificial sweetener

A little dried parsley, for garnishing

Serves 1
Carbohydrates: 2 g

51

Sliced aubergine and Mozzarella grill

Based on a classic Italian dish, this makes a sensational lunch. Slices of aubergine, smeared with olive oil, topped with tomato, basil and melting Mozzarella, then grilled.

½ aubergine (eggplant)

15 ml/1 tbsp olive oil

15 ml/1 tbsp tomato purée (paste)

1.5 ml/¼ tsp dried basil

Freshly ground black pepper

50 g/2 oz/½ cup grated Mozzarella cheese

1 Cut the aubergine lengthways into three slices. Brush the slices all over with the olive oil.

2 Place on foil on a grill (broiler) rack. Cook under a preheated grill (broiler) for about 3 minutes on each side until golden and cooked through.

3 Gently spread the tomato purée over the slices. Sprinkle with the basil and pepper and top with the cheese.

4 Return to the grill for about 2–3 minutes until the cheese is bubbling and just turning golden in places. Serve straight away.

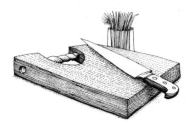

Serves 1

Carbohydrates: 11 g

Button mushroom and chive omelette

A simple lunch that will really tempt the taste buds. A soft, golden omelette enveloping sliced button mushrooms, gently cooked and flavoured with fresh, snipped chives.

1 Put the mushrooms in a pan with half the water. Bring to the boil, reduce the heat and simmer gently for 3–4 minutes until cooked through. If necessary, turn up the heat and boil rapidly, stirring, to remove any remaining liquid. Alternatively, microwave the mushrooms with just 15 ml/1 tbsp of water for 2 minutes on Full Power.

2 Whisk the eggs with the remaining 30 ml/2 tbsp water, a pinch of salt and a good grinding of pepper.

3 Melt the butter in an omelette pan. Add the eggs and cook, lifting and stirring as the mixture begins to set, to allow the uncooked egg to run underneath.

4 When the omelette is partially set and beginning to turn golden underneath, spoon the mushrooms over half the surface and sprinkle with the chives. Cook for a further 2 minutes until the base is golden and the egg is just set but still creamy. Fold the plain side of the omelette over the mushroom half, then slide on to a plate.

50 g/2 oz button mushrooms, sliced

60 ml/4 tbsp water

2 eggs

Salt and freshly ground black pepper

15 g/½ oz/1 tbsp butter

15 ml/1 tbsp snipped fresh chives

Serves 1
Carbohydrates: Trace

Avocado with prawns in Thousand Island dressing

Sometimes you simply can't beat the classics. But in this case you can have a whole *avocado, filled with succulent prawns and topped with your favourite pink seafood mayonnaise!*

1 avocado

A squeeze of lemon juice

A good handful of shredded lettuce

5 slices of cucumber

60 ml/4 tbsp cooked peeled prawns (shrimp)

15 ml/1 tbsp mayonnaise

5 ml/1 tsp tomato purée (paste)

15 ml/1 tbsp double (heavy) cream

2.5 ml/½ tsp Worcestershire sauce

Freshly ground black pepper

A pinch of cayenne

A wedge of lemon, for garnishing

1 Cut the avocado in half and remove the stone (pit). Brush the cut surfaces with lemon juice.

2 Put the lettuce in a shallow dish, set the avocado halves on top and arrange the cucumber slices around.

3 Pile the prawns into the cavities in the avocado halves.

4 Mix the mayonnaise with the tomato purée, cream, Worcestershire sauce and a good grinding of pepper. Stir in the cayenne.

5 Spoon the sauce over the prawns and garnish with a wedge of lemon.

Serves 1
Carbohydrates: 8 g

Chilled cream of cucumber soup with dill

Cool, refreshing and revitalising – just three adjectives to describe this delicious soup, which makes a perfect lunch dish, especially on a hot day.

1 Coarsely grate the cucumber into a colander. Sprinkle well with salt and leave to stand for 10 minutes. Rinse with cold water, then squeeze out all the moisture.

2 Tip the cucumber into a bowl and stir in the dill, vinegar and crème fraîche.

3 Stir in a good grinding of pepper, then chill, if time allows.

4 When ready to serve, stir in the cold water, taste and adjust the seasoning, if necessary.

7.5 cm/3 in piece of cucumber

Salt

2.5 ml/½ tsp dried dill (dill weed)

7.5 ml/1½ tsp white wine vinegar

75 ml/5 tbsp crème fraîche

Freshly ground black pepper

75 ml/5 tbsp cold water

Serves 1
Carbohydrates: 4 g

55

Grilled chicken legs in lemon and garlic marinade

Marinating imparts flavour and tenderness, but do allow time for the flavours to penetrate. You can cook these one day to serve the next or make a larger quantity to keep in the fridge.

3 chicken legs

30 ml/2 tbsp olive oil

5 ml/1 tsp lemon juice

A good pinch of garlic salt

1 slice of onion, separated into rings

1.5 ml/¼ tsp dried oregano or rosemary

Freshly ground black pepper

1 Wipe the chicken legs with kitchen paper (paper towels).

2 Mix the remaining ingredients together in a shallow ovenproof dish, just large enough to take the legs in one layer. Put the chicken in the dish, turning over in the marinade to coat completely. Cover and chill to marinate for at least 3 hours, turning occasionally.

3 Remove the onion rings, then roast the chicken in a preheated oven at 190°C/375°F/gas 5/fan oven 170°C for about 30 minutes, turning once, until golden and cooked through. Alternatively cook under a preheated grill (broiler), basting with the marinade and turning occasionally, for 20–25 minutes until cooked through.

4 Serve hot or cold.

Serves 1

Carbohydrates: 0 g

Lettuce and cucumber rolls with Cheddar

A clever idea for a cool tempting light meal, this dish uses lettuce instead of bread as the wrap around a cheese, mayonnaise and cucumber filling.

1 Mix the cheese with the mayonnaise.

2 Lay the lettuce leaves on a board, undersides up. Spread with the cheese mixture.

3 Lay the cucumber sticks in the centre of one edge of each leaf. Fold in the sides, then roll up so that the shiny upper side of the leaf is on the outside.

40 g/1½ oz/⅓ cup grated Cheddar cheese

60 ml/4 tbsp mayonnaise

3 large lettuce leaves

5 cm/2 in piece of cucumber, cut into very thin matchsticks

Serves 1
Carbohydrates: 3 g

Ham, cheese and asparagus rolls

A simple way with three favourite ingredients – sweet-cured ham, cool, creamy white cheese and asparagus spears – all rolled into one tasty lunch dish.

1 Lay the ham on a board and spread thinly with the cheese. Season with pepper.

2 Drain the spears and divide between the ham slices, laying them along one edge, then roll up.

3 slices of lean ham

25 g/1 oz/1 tbsp of cream cheese

Freshly ground black pepper

½ x 300 g/11 oz/ medium can of asparagus spears

Serves 1
Carbohydrates: 1 g

Dinner Recipes

These meals will leave you feeling satisfied and thoroughly pampered. Enjoy every morsel and don't forget to eat your dessert, too. If you don't like a particular vegetable, swap it for another of the same carbohydrate value. You can, of course, simply grill, fry or poach – as appropriate – the meat, poultry or fish and serve it with all the vegetables plainly cooked. The carbohydrate count won't alter, but the calorie count might!

All the recipes in this section are designed for one, but they are delicious enough to serve to the whole family.

Moreish and golden celeriac chips

These are an ingenious alternative to potato chips - something low-carb dieters often miss! They taste superb and, of course, they are incredibly low in carbohydrates.

¼ celeriac (celery root), peeled and cut into thick fingers

Oil, for cooking

1 Cook the celeriac in boiling water for 2 minutes. Drain well.

2 Heat about 2 cm/¾ in of oil in a frying pan (skillet). Add the celeriac and cook for about 3 minutes, turning occasionally, until golden brown. Drain on kitchen paper (paper towels).

3 Serve hot.

Serves 1
Carbohydrates: 3 g

Sirloin steak with mushrooms in garlic butter

A succulent steak with garlic mushrooms, fresh green broccoli and sweet baby corn cobs. Prepare the celeriac for the chips in advance and fry them when cooking the other vegetables.

1 Season the steak with salt and pepper. Place on foil on a grill (broiler) rack and dot with a quarter of the butter.

2 Melt two-thirds of the remaining butter in a small pan. Add the mushrooms and garlic, cover and cook for about 4 minutes over a gentle heat, shaking the pan occasionally, until cooked through. Keep warm.

3 Grill (broil) the steak for 2–3 minutes on one side until golden. Turn over and dot with the remaining butter. Grill for a further 2–6 minutes, depending on how well you like your steak cooked.

4 Add the broccoli to a pan of boiling water and cook for 1 minute. Add the corn cobs and cook for a further 3 minutes until tender. Drain.

5 Transfer the steak to a warm plate and top with the garlic mushrooms. Serve with the broccoli, corn cobs and Celeriac Chips.

1 sirloin steak, about 175 g/6 oz

Salt and freshly ground black pepper

25 g/1 oz/2 tbsp butter

6 button mushrooms

½ small garlic clove, crushed

15 ml/1 tbsp chopped fresh parsley

4 medium broccoli florets

4 baby corn cobs

Serve with:

Celeriac Chips (see page 58)

Serves 1

Carbohydrates: 8 g (including 3 g for the Celeriac Chips)

Greek aubergine moussaka

This is a great recipe that all the family will want to share. If so, you can easily make a larger quantity and cook it in a bigger dish. The cooking time will be much the same.

30 ml/2 tbsp olive oil

½ aubergine (eggplant), sliced

½ small onion, chopped

100 g/4 oz minced (ground) lamb

5 ml/1 tsp tomato purée (paste)

60 ml/4 tbsp water

A good pinch each of ground cinnamon and dried oregano

Salt and freshly ground black pepper

1 small egg, beaten

60 ml/4 tbsp crème fraîche

15 g/½ oz/2 tbsp grated Cheddar cheese

Serve with:

Lamb's Tongue Lettuce and Radish Salad (see page 61)

Serves 1

Carbohydrates: 10 g (including 2 g for the salad)

1 Heat 20 ml/4 tsp of the oil in a frying pan (skillet). Fry (sauté) the aubergine slices until golden on both sides. Drain on kitchen paper (paper towels).

2 Heat the remaining oil in a saucepan. Add the onion and lamb and cook, stirring, until the lamb is no longer pink and all the grains are separate.

3 Stir in the tomato purée, water, cinnamon and oregano. Season to taste with salt and pepper. Simmer, stirring occasionally, for 5 minutes.

4 Layer the meat and aubergine slices in an individual ovenproof dish, finishing with a layer of aubergine.

5 Whisk the egg and crème fraîche together with a good grinding of pepper. Stir in the cheese and spoon over the aubergine layer.

6 Bake in a preheated oven at 190°C/ 375°F/gas 5/fan oven 170°C for about 35 minutes until the top is golden and set. Meanwhile, make the salad.

7 Serve the moussaka hot or at room temperature with the salad.

Lamb's tongue lettuce and radish salad

Tender-sweet lamb's tongue lettuce (also known as corn salad), blended with slightly peppery pink radishes, fresh chives and plump green olives, simply dressed with oil and vinegar.

1 Put the lettuce on a flat plate and scatter the radish slices and chives over. Trickle with the oil and vinegar, then season well with pepper.

2 Scatter the olives over and serve.

A good handful of lamb's tongue lettuce

5 radishes, sliced

15 ml/1 tbsp snipped fresh chives

15 ml/1 tbsp olive oil

5 ml/1 tsp red wine vinegar

Freshly ground black pepper

5 green olives

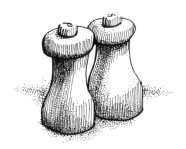

Serves 1

Carbohydrates: 2 g

Grilled cheese-topped gammon with courgettes

A nutty-sweet, melting cheese is the ideal topping for a juicy tender gammon steak and is perfectly accompanied by young French beans and sautéed courgettes.

1 gammon steak

100 g/4 oz French (green) beans, topped and tailed

15 ml/1 tbsp olive oil

1 medium courgette (zucchini), sliced

Freshly ground black pepper

2 slices of Havarti or Emmental (Swiss) cheese

1 Snip all round the edge of the gammon steak with scissors to stop it curling when cooked. Place it on the grill (broiler) rack and cook under a preheated grill for about 3 minutes on each side until golden and cooked through.

2 Meanwhile, cook the beans in boiling, lightly salted water for 4–5 minutes until just tender. Drain.

3 Heat the oil in a frying pan (skillet) and fry (sauté) the courgette slices, turning occasionally, for 3–4 minutes until golden and cooked through. Drain on kitchen paper (paper towels) and season with pepper.

4 Lay the slices of cheese on top of the cooked gammon and return to the grill until melted and bubbling.

5 Transfer the gammon steak to a warm plate. Spoon the courgettes and beans to one side and serve.

Serves 1

Carbohydrates: 8 g

Warm salmon salad with asparagus

A sophisticated salad of chicory, lettuce and watercress, garnished with tomatoes and cucumber and delicately cooked asparagus, topped with grilled salmon and a creamy dressing.

1 Trim and discard the hard base of the asparagus stalks. Cook the spears in a little boiling, lightly salted water for 3 minutes only. Turn off the heat and leave to stand for 5 minutes, then drain, rinse and drain again.

2 Cut a cone-shaped core out of the base of the chicory, then separate into leaves and cut into chunks. Trim the feathery stalks off the watercress, then tear into manageable pieces. Mix the lettuce, chicory and watercress on a plate and arrange the asparagus spears on the top. Scatter the tomatoes and cucumber over too.

3 Put the salmon on a piece of foil under a preheated grill (broiler), skin-side down, and grill (broil) for about 6 minutes until lightly golden and just cooked. The exact time will depend on the thickness but take care not to overcook it. Place on top of the salad.

4 Whisk the oil with the lemon juice and mayonnaise. Thin with the water and season well with pepper.

5 Spoon the dressing over the salmon so that it trickles down over the salad.

---

10 short thin asparagus spears

1 head of chicory (Belgian endive)

A good handful of roughly torn iceberg lettuce

A good handful of watercress

4 cherry tomatoes, quartered

2.5 cm/1 in piece of cucumber, diced

1 piece of salmon tail fillet, about 175 g/6 oz

10 ml/2 tsp olive oil

5 ml/1 tsp lemon juice

15 ml/1 tbsp mayonnaise

15 ml/1 tbsp water

Freshly ground black pepper

Serves 1
Carbohydrates: 8 g

Pan-roasted chicken with mushrooms and turnips

Sautéed chicken, mushrooms and turnips, subtly flavoured with garlic and fresh parsley, then served with all the rich, buttery pan juices poured over the top.

15 g/½ oz/1 tbsp butter

15 ml/1 tbsp olive oil

1 chicken leg portion

4 baby turnips, halved

50 g/2 oz button mushrooms

Salt and freshly ground black pepper

75 ml/5 tbsp chicken stock, made with ¼ stock cube

10 ml/2 tsp fresh chopped parsley

½ small garlic clove, chopped

Serve with:

Fresh Green Salad with Rocket and Basil (see page 65)

Serves 1

Carbohydrates: 5 g (including 2 g for the salad)

1 Heat half the butter and half the oil in a frying pan (skillet). Add the chicken and fry (sauté) for about 5 minutes until browned all over. Remove from the pan.

2 Add the remaining butter and oil and fry the turnips for 2–3 minutes, stirring and turning until lightly golden.

3 Return the chicken to the pan and add the mushrooms. Season lightly with salt and pepper. Turn down the heat, cover the pan with a lid or foil and cook gently for 30 minutes until the chicken and turnips are tender.

4 Sprinkle the parsley and garlic over, re-cover and cook for a further 5 minutes.

5 Make the salad.

6 Remove the chicken and vegetables from the pan and keep warm.

7 Pour the stock into the pan and boil, stirring, until slightly reduced. Spoon over the chicken and serve with the salad.

Fresh green salad with rocket and basil

A simple, fresh crisp salad is the perfect low-carbohydrate accompaniment to almost any meal. You could use watercress or a head of chicory instead of rocket.

1 Put the lettuce, rocket, cucumber and spring onion in a bowl.

2 Whisk the remaining ingredients together and pour over. Toss gently.

A good handful of torn lettuce leaves

A good handful of rocket

5 slices of cucumber

1 spring onion (scallion), chopped

2–3 fresh basil leaves, torn

15 ml/1 tbsp olive oil

5 ml/1 tsp red wine vinegar

A pinch of artificial sweetener

Salt and freshly ground black pepper

1.5 ml/¼ tsp Dijon mustard

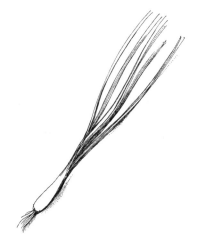

Serves 1

Carbohydrates: 2 g

Lamb shank with rosemary jus

Meltingly tender garlic-flavoured lamb served with the reduced meat juices lifted with rosemary and blackcurrant. The Celeriac and Carrot Mash adds an extra gourmet touch.

1 large sprig of fresh rosemary, plus a small sprig for garnishing

1 lamb shank

½ small garlic clove, cut into slivers

150 ml/¼ pt/⅔ cup lamb or chicken stock, made with ¼ stock cube

10 ml/2 tsp undiluted sugar-free real blackcurrant cordial

Salt and freshly ground black pepper

Serve with:

Creamy Celeriac and Carrot Mash (see page 67) and Peppery Wild Rocket Salad (see page 67)

Serves 1

Carbohydrates: 9 g (including 9 g for the Celeriac and Carrot Mash)

1 Put the large sprig of rosemary in a small casserole dish (Dutch oven). Lay the lamb on top. Make a few small cuts in the flesh with a sharp-pointed knife and insert a sliver of garlic into each.

2 Pour the stock around and add the cordial. Sprinkle the meat with salt and pepper.

3 Cook in a preheated oven at 160°C/ 325°F/gas 3/fan oven 145°C for 2½–3 hours until meltingly tender.

4 When the lamb is nearly cooked, make the mash and the salad.

5 Lift the lamb out of the casserole and keep warm. Discard the rosemary.

6 Spoon off any fat floating on the surface. Boil the juices rapidly until reduced and syrupy. Taste and re-season, if necessary.

7 Serve the lamb on a pile of Celeriac and Carrot Mash and spoon the jus over. Garnish with a small sprig of rosemary and serve with the salad.

Creamy celeriac and carrot mash

A wonderful alternative to potato mash - whether or not potatoes are forbidden! - this delicious dish is high in fibre and sumptuous in flavour.

1 Cut the celeriac into small chunks. Boil the celeriac and carrot together in lightly salted water for about 8–10 minutes until tender. Drain well.

2 Mash thoroughly with the butter and beat in a good grinding of pepper.

¼ small celeriac (celery root)

1 carrot, sliced

A knob of butter

Serves 1
Carbohydrates: 9 g

Peppery wild rocket salad

Peppery, fresh rocket makes a great accompaniment to most main courses, especially grilled meats. Here it is dressed with olive oil, red wine vinegar and just a hint of herbs.

1 Put the rocket in a bowl.

2 Whisk the remaining ingredients together and trickle over. Toss gently.

1 good handful of rocket

10 ml/2 tsp olive oil

4 ml/¾ tsp red wine vinegar

A good pinch of dried mixed herbs

A pinch of artificial sweetener

Salt and freshly ground black pepper

Serves 1
Carbohydrates: Trace

Roast pork with swede and roasted onions

It's not worth cooking this mouth-watering roast for one. If you are eating alone, cook a quarter of the vegetables with the joint, then eat the remaining pork at any meal – it has no carbs at all.

1 small swede (rutabaga), cut into large chunks

1 kg/2¼ lb piece of leg of pork, with crackling

30 ml/2 tbsp olive oil

Salt

4 onions, halved

For the gravy:

1 pork or chicken stock cube

2.5 ml/½ tsp dried sage

15 ml/1 tbsp undiluted sugar-free real blackcurrant cordial

Freshly ground black pepper

Serve with:

Mangetout (snow peas)

Serves 4

Carbohydrates: 13 g per serving (including 3 g for the mangetout)

1 Boil the swede in lightly salted water for 2 minutes. Drain, reserving the water.

2 Score the pork rind, then rub with a little of the oil and some salt. Place the joint on a trivet in the centre of a roasting tin (pan).

3 Toss the swede and onions in the rest of the oil and arrange round the pork.

4 Roast in a preheated oven at 220°C/ 425°F/gas 7/fan oven 200°C for 30 minutes. Turn down the heat to 190°C/375°F/gas 5/fan oven 170°C and roast for a further hour, turning the swede and onions after 30 minutes.

5 Transfer the meat and vegetables to a carving dish and keep warm. Spoon off any excess fat from the roasting tin, but leave all the meat juices.

6 Pour 450 ml/¾ pt/2 cups of the swede cooking water into the roasting tin. Crumble in the stock cube and add the sage and blackcurrant cordial. Boil rapidly, scraping up any sediment, for 5 minutes until slightly reduced. Season with pepper.

7 Carve as much of the pork as you want and serve with the roast swede and onions, the mangetout and gravy.

Chicken and bamboo shoots with pak choi

An exciting stir-fry of tender strips of chicken, mushrooms, spring onions, bamboo shoots and shredded green pak choi, tossed in soy sauce and lightly flavoured with Chinese spices.

1 Heat the oil in a frying pan (skillet) or wok. Add the chicken and stir-fry for 3 minutes.

2 Add the spring onions and stir-fry for 2 minutes.

3 Add the bamboo shoots, pak choi and mushrooms and stir-fry for 4 minutes until everything is just cooked.

4 Stir in the soy sauce, water and five-spice powder.

5 Toss well before serving.

15 ml/1 tbsp sunflower oil

1 skinless chicken breast, cut into thin strips

4 spring onions (scallions), cut diagonally into 5 cm/ 2 in lengths

½ x 225 g/8 oz/small can of bamboo shoots, drained

1 head of pak choi, shredded

4 mushrooms, sliced

5 ml/1 tsp soy sauce

5 ml/1 tsp water

A pinch of Chinese five-spice powder

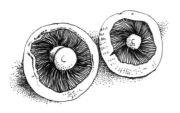

Serves 1
Carbohydrates: 4 g

Liver, bacon and savoy with onion gravy

Meltingly moist slices of liver served with bacon rashers on a bed of shredded, lightly cooked cabbage, bathed in onion gravy. Cook the Crushed Swede when you start to boil the cabbage (Step 4).

1 onion, chopped

15 g/½ oz/1 tbsp butter

120 ml/4 fl oz/½ cup beef stock, made with ¼ stock cube

15 ml/1 tbsp sunflower or olive oil

3 rashers (slices) of back bacon, rinded

100 g/4 oz/small wedge of Savoy cabbage, stalk removed and shredded

3 medium slices of lambs' liver

Salt and freshly ground black pepper

Serve with:

Crushed Swede with Butter and Cream (see page 71)

Serves 1

Carbohydrates: 14 g (including 2 g for the Crushed Swede)

1 Fry (sauté) the onion in the butter, stirring, for 4 minutes until golden.

2 Add the stock, bring to the boil and boil rapidly for several minutes until well reduced and slightly syrupy.

3 Heat the oil in a frying pan (skillet) and fry the bacon on both sides until golden. Remove from the pan.

4 Meanwhile, cook the cabbage in a small pan with about 2.5 cm/1 in of boiling, lightly salted water, stirring once or twice, for 3 minutes until just tender but still with some 'bite'. Drain, reserving the cooking water.

5 Season the liver well with pepper, add to the pan and fry for 2–3 minutes on one side until golden. Turn over and fry just until droplets of blood rise to the surface. Remove from the pan and keep warm.

6 Put the onion mixture in the frying pan and add the cabbage cooking water. Stir well, bring to the boil and boil rapidly for 1–2 minutes until slightly thickened. Season to taste.

7 Pile the cabbage on a warm plate, top with the liver and bacon, spoon the gravy over. Serve with Crushed Swede.

Crushed swede with butter and cream

A golden-pink, well-flavoured mound of softly cooked swede, blended with cream and butter and spiked with black pepper. It makes a great alternative to potatoes.

1 Cut the swede into small chunks and boil in lightly salted water for 8–10 minutes until tender. Drain and return to the pan.

2 Cook over a gentle heat for 1–2 minutes to dry out.

3 Add a good grinding of pepper, then mash thoroughly with the cream and butter.

¼ small swede (rutabaga)

Salt and freshly ground black pepper

15 ml/1 tbsp double (heavy) cream

A small knob of butter

Serves 1

Carbohydrates: 2 g

Garlic-sautéed courgettes

One of the best ways of cooking courgettes, this really enhances their flavour. It is delicious with grilled tuna, or can be served with other meat or fish dishes.

1 Melt the butter in a frying pan (skillet). Add the courgettes, garlic and a good grinding of pepper.

2 Cook over a fairly high heat for about 6 minutes, stirring and turning the slices as necessary, until golden brown on both sides.

3 Drain on kitchen paper (paper towels), if liked, or serve in their buttery juices.

15 g/½ oz/1 tbsp butter

2 small courgettes (zucchini), sliced

½ small garlic clove, crushed

Freshly ground black pepper

Serves 1

Carbohydrates: 4 g

Grilled tuna with peppers and olives

A juicy steak of meaty fish, flavoured with the subtle, smoky flavour of Spanish pimentón, cooked until just pink and served with colourful grilled peppers, scattered with stuffed olives.

1 tuna steak, about 175 g/6 oz

20 ml/4 tsp olive oil

2.5 ml/½ tsp sweet pimentón

Salt and freshly ground black pepper

1 green (bell) pepper, cut into thick strips

1 yellow pepper, cut into thick strips

5 ml/1 tsp fresh chopped parsley

6 stuffed olives, sliced

Serve with:

Garlic-sautéed Courgettes (see page 71)

1 Brush the tuna with a little of the oil and season on both sides with the pimentón, a very little salt and lots of black pepper.

2 Toss the pepper strips in the remaining oil and arrange on foil on a grill (broiler) rack. Cook under a preheated grill (broiler) for 4 minutes. Turn over and put the tuna alongside.

3 Grill (broil) for 2 minutes. Turn the tuna over and rearrange any pepper slices so that they can brown evenly. Grill for a further 2–4 minutes until the fish is just cooked but slightly pink in the centre and the peppers are browning at the edges.

4 Transfer to a warm plate with any juices. Sprinkle the tuna with parsley and scatter the olives over the peppers.

5 Serve with Garlic-sautéed Courgettes.

Serves 1

Carbohydrates: 15 g (including 4 g for the Garlic-sautéed Courgettes)

Warm smoked haddock and quails' egg salad

A sensational salad of golden smoked haddock, tiny quails' eggs and crisp Italian bacon on a bed of baby spinach, bathed in a warm dressing of olive oil, crème fraîche and red wine vinegar.

1 Put the fish in a shallow pan and cover with water. Put the quails' eggs alongside. Bring to the boil, boil for just 30 seconds for soft-boiled eggs or exactly 3 minutes for hard-boiled (hard-cooked), then quickly remove the eggs and put them in a bowl of cold water to prevent further cooking.

2 Cover the pan and poach the fish for a further 5 minutes or until tender. Drain. Remove the skin and cut the fish into bite-sized pieces.

3 Dry-fry the pancetta in a frying pan (skillet), stirring until crisp. Remove from the pan and drain on kitchen paper (paper towels).

4 Pile the spinach on a plate and scatter the pancetta, fish, tomatoes, cucumber and chives over.

5 Shell and halve the eggs and arrange around, taking care if they are soft-boiled as the yolks will be runny.

6 Put the oil and vinegar in the pan with the pancetta fat and bring to the boil, stirring. Stir in the crème fraîche and season with sweetener, salt and lots of pepper. Spoon over the salad.

1 piece of smoked haddock fillet, about 175 g/6 oz

4 quails' eggs, scrubbed

50 g/2 oz diced pancetta

2 good handfuls of baby spinach leaves

2 cherry tomatoes, quartered

2.5 cm/1 in piece of cucumber, diced

15 ml/1 tbsp snipped fresh chives

30 ml/2 tbsp olive oil

10 ml/2 tsp red wine vinegar

10 ml/2 tsp crème fraîche

A pinch of artificial sweetener

Salt and freshly ground black pepper

Serves 1

Carbohydrates: 4 g

Grilled mackerel with mustard rub

The mustard rub brings out all the flavour and succulence of fresh mackerel. Fresh runner beans offset the richness of the fish. Prepare the Scalloped Carrots before you cook the beans (Step 4).

1.5 ml/¼ tsp mustard powder

1.5 ml/¼ tsp dried oregano

1.5 ml/¼ tsp paprika

1.5 ml/¼ tsp onion salt

A good pinch of artificial sweetener

Freshly ground black pepper

1 large mackerel, cleaned

A little oil, for greasing

100 g/4 oz runner beans

Serve with:

Scalloped Carrots with Fresh Coriander (see page 75)

Serves 1

Carbohydrates: 10 g (including 8 g for the Scalloped Carrots)

1 Mix the mustard powder with the oregano, paprika, onion salt, sweetener and a good grinding of pepper.

2 Rinse the mackerel and dry with kitchen paper (paper towels). Cut off the head, if liked. Make several slashes in the body on both sides.

3 Rub the mustard mixture into the slits in the mackerel, then chill for at least 2 hours to let the flavours to develop.

4 When ready to cook, string the beans and cut them diagonally into slices. Bring a small pan of lightly salted water to the boil, add the beans and cook for about 4 minutes until just tender. Drain and keep warm.

5 While the vegetables are cooking, preheat the grill (broiler). Oil the rack, then put the mackerel on it and grill (broil) for 4–5 minutes until golden. Turn over and cook the other side for 4–5 minutes until golden brown and cooked through.

6 Transfer the mackerel to a warm plate and serve with the runner beans and Scalloped Carrots.

Scalloped carrots with fresh coriander

For this unusual and delicious way of serving carrots, you simmer the sliced vegetables in buttery juices with a little chopped fresh coriander.

1 Heat the butter in a small frying pan (skillet). Add the carrot slices and toss well to coat.

2 Sprinkle with salt, pepper and the sweetener and add the water. Cover with a lid or foil and cook over a gentle heat for 10 minutes, stirring once or twice, until tender.

3 Remove the lid or foil and boil rapidly, if necessary, to remove any excess liquid. The carrots should be moist but not wet. Stir in the coriander just before serving.

15 g/½ oz/1 tbsp butter

1 large carrot, cut diagonally into thin slices

Salt and freshly ground black pepper

A pinch of artificial sweetener

45 ml/3 tbsp water

5 ml/1 tsp chopped fresh coriander (cilantro)

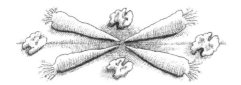

Serves 1
Carbohydrates: 8 g

Peppered pork chop with sautéed caraway cabbage

A juicy chop coated in freshly crushed peppercorns, seared until tender and served with shredded white cabbage, lightly fried in olive oil and butter and subtly flavoured with caraway seeds.

1 lean pork chop, about 175 g/6 oz

5 ml/1 tsp coarsely crushed black peppercorns

15 g/½ oz/1 tbsp butter

15 ml/1 tbsp olive oil

100 g/4 oz wedge of white cabbage, stalk removed and shredded

2.5 ml/½ tsp caraway seeds

Salt

90 ml/6 tbsp chicken or vegetable stock, made with ¼ stock cube

Serve with:

Okra Provençale with Spring Onions and Garlic (see page 77)

Serves 1

Carbohydrates: 11 g (including 8 g for the Okra Provençale)

1 Coat the pork chop in the peppercorns on both sides.

2 Heat half the butter and half the oil in a frying pan (skillet). Add the shredded cabbage and caraway seeds and fry (sauté), stirring, for about 5 minutes until lightly golden and just tender. Season with a tiny sprinkling of salt, remove from the pan with a draining spoon and keep warm.

3 Heat the remaining oil in the pan. Add the pork and fry quickly for 2 minutes on each side to brown. Turn down the heat and cook more gently for a further 15–20 minutes until cooked right through.

4 Lift the pork out of the pan and keep warm. Pour in the stock and boil, scraping up any sediment in the bottom of the pan for 1 minute. Whisk in the remaining butter, a little at a time, to thicken the sauce, then season with a little salt, if liked.

5 Put the sautéed cabbage on a warm plate. Top with the pork and spoon the gravy over. Serve with Okra Provençale.

Okra Provençale
with spring onions and garlic

This sensational accompaniment of fingers of okra, bathed in a rich tomato, spring onion and garlic sauce, is also delicious made with courgettes.

1 Boil the okra in lightly salted water for 5 minutes until almost tender. Drain well.

2 Heat the oil in a small saucepan. Add the spring onions and garlic and fry (sauté) for 2 minutes, stirring. Add the tomatoes, tomato purée and water, bring to the boil and boil for 2 minutes until pulpy.

3 Add the okra, a little salt and pepper and the artificial sweetener. Cover and simmer for 2–3 minutes, stirring occasionally, until the okra is bathed in sauce.

4 Serve hot.

100 g/4 oz okra (ladies' fingers)

5 ml/1 tsp olive oil

1 spring onion (scallion), chopped

½ small garlic clove, crushed

2 ripe tomatoes, skinned and chopped

2.5 ml/½ tsp tomato purée (paste)

30 ml/2 tbsp water

Salt and freshly ground black pepper

A pinch of artificial sweetener

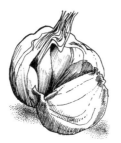

Serves 1
Carbohydrates: 8 g

Beef Stroganoff with mushrooms and brandy

Strips of the tenderest beef quickly cooked with mushrooms and onion, bathed in a crème fraîche sauce laced with brandy. It is best to start cooking the Broccoli and Cauliflower Sauté first.

1 small onion, sliced

4 button mushrooms, sliced

100 g/4 oz fillet steak, cut into thin strips

Salt and freshly ground black pepper

10 ml/2 tsp brandy (optional)

75 ml/5 tbsp crème fraîche

10 ml/2 tsp chopped fresh parsley

Serve with:

Broccoli and Cauliflower Sauté (see page 79)

1 Fry (sauté) the onion and mushrooms in the butter for 3 minutes, stirring, until softened but only lightly golden.

2 Add the steak and continue to stir-fry for 3–4 minutes until the steak is just cooked.

3 Season well, then pour over the brandy, if using, and ignite. Shake the pan until the flames subside, then stir in the crème fraîche and parsley. Simmer for about 2 minutes until slightly thickened. Taste and re-season, if necessary.

4 Serve with Broccoli and Cauliflower Sauté.

Serves 1

Carbohydrates: 13 g (including 5 g for the Broccoli and Cauliflower Sauté)

Broccoli and cauliflower sauté

A perfect accompaniment to beef, this dish is made up of tiny florets of broccoli and cauliflower tossed in olive oil with fragrant coriander seeds and just a hint of garlic.

1 Heat the oil in a frying pan (skillet). Add the cauliflower and broccoli and fry (sauté) for 2 minutes, stirring.

2 Add the coriander, garlic, a few grains of salt and lots of pepper. Cook, stirring, for about 5 minutes until just tender and slightly golden round the edges.

15 ml/1 tbsp olive oil

¼ small cauliflower, cut into 8 tiny florets

100 g/4 oz broccoli, cut into 8 tiny florets

2.5 ml/½ tsp coriander (cilantro) seeds, crushed

½ small garlic clove, crushed

Salt and freshly ground black pepper

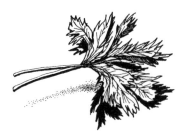

Serves 1
Carbohydrates: 5 g

Desserts and Savouries for Lunch and Dinner

These recipes offer perfect ways to round off all your meals. When sugar-free jelly is called for, simply make it according to the packet directions and eat as much as you like!

Venetian coffee cream cheese

You can make this smooth, bitter-sweet dessert in advance and leave it to chill while you prepare your meal. Serve it very cold to offset the richness of the flavour.

4 ml/³⁄₄ tsp instant coffee granules

5 ml/1 tsp boiling water

50 g/2 oz/¹⁄₄ cup cream cheese

Artificial sweetener, to taste

1 Dissolve the coffee in the water in a small bowl.

2 Beat in the cheese and sweeten to taste.

3 Pile in a small glass serving dish and chill until ready to serve.

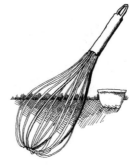

Serves 1
Carbohydrates: Trace

Refreshing summer fruit frostie

So simple and so refreshing to enjoy at any time, this is easy to make for one, or you can increase the quantities and leave some in the freezer to take out servings as you want them.

1 Mix the cordial with the water (it should taste quite strong). Pour into a shallow freezer-proof container. Freeze for about 1½ hours or until firm around the edges.

2 Whisk with a fork thoroughly to break up the ice crystals, then freeze again until just frozen.

3 When ready to serve, tip the flavoured ice out into a bowl and whisk with a fork until slushy, then serve. If very hard, tip into a blender or food processor and run the machine briefly until the mixture becomes soft and slushy.

30 ml/2 tbsp no-calorie summer fruit cordial

150 ml/¼ pt/⅔ cup water

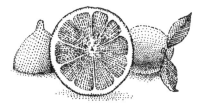

Serves 1
Carbohydrates: 0 g

Rhubarb with creamy custard sauce

It's not possible to make just one portion of custard, so I've made enough of this dessert for two. Either share it or store the second portion in the fridge and serve in place of another 2-carb dessert.

225 g/8 oz rhubarb, cut into short lengths

60 ml/4 tbsp water

Artificial sweetener, to taste

For the custard:

75 ml/5 tbsp double (heavy) cream

75 ml/5 tbsp water

1 egg

1.5 ml/¼ tsp vanilla essence (extract)

15 ml/1 tbsp artificial sweetener

1 Put the rhubarb in a saucepan with the water. Bring to the boil, turn down the heat and cook very gently for about 10 minutes until tender. Don't boil rapidly or the rhubarb will fall to a pulp. Sweeten to taste.

2 Meanwhile, mix the cream and water together in a saucepan and heat until hot but not boiling. Whisk the egg and vanilla together in a bowl.

3 Whisk in the hot cream and water. Put the bowl over a saucepan of gently simmering water and stir frequently with a wooden spoon until the custard is thick enough to just coat the back of the spoon (this may take up to 15 minutes). Stir in the sweetener.

4 Serve the custard and rhubarb hot or cold.

Serves 2

Carbohydrates: 2 g per serving

Grilled avocado slices with crème fraîche

Slices of creamy-smooth avocado, brushed with butter and flavoured with lime or lemon before being lightly grilled, sweetened and served with crème fraîche.

1 Peel the avocado and cut into slices. Place on a grill (broiler) rack.

2 Melt the butter with the lime or lemon zest and brush all over the avocado slices.

3 Grill (broil) for about 3 minutes until turning slightly golden.

4 Transfer the slices to a warm plate and sprinkle with a little artificial sweetener, if liked.

5 Serve with a spoonful of crème fraîche.

½ small ripe avocado, stoned (pitted)

A knob of butter

Finely grated zest of ¼ lime or ¼ small lemon

A pinch of artificial sweetener (optional)

15 ml/1 tbsp crème fraîche

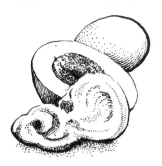

Serves 1
Carbohydrates: 1 g

Rum and chocolate mousse

A one-egg quantity is just too much for one serving, so I suggest you chill the remainder of this delicious mousse for another day instead of another 2-carb dessert – or share it with a friend!

10 ml/2 tsp cocoa (unsweetened chocolate) powder

15 ml/1 tbsp boiling water

15 ml/1 tbsp artificial sweetener

1.5 ml/¼ tsp rum essence (extract)

1 egg, separated

60 ml/4 tbsp double (heavy) cream

1 Blend the cocoa with the boiling water and sweetener and stir until smooth. Stir in the rum essence and whisk in the egg yolk.

2 Whisk the egg white until stiff. Whisk the cream separately until peaking. Fold the cream into the cocoa mixture, then finally fold in the egg white. Taste and add more rum essence, if liked.

3 Turn into a small serving dish and chill until firm.

Serves 2
Carbohydrates: 2 g

Light and creamy mocha whip

A coffee-chocolate fluffy dessert with a dash of cream. Store the egg yolk covered with water in a small container in the fridge. You can use it for Baked Vanilla Cream (see page 88).

1 Dissolve the coffee and cocoa in the water and stir in the sweetener.

2 Whisk the egg white until stiff, and whip the cream separately until peaking.

3 Gently whisk the mocha mixture into the cream, then fold in the egg white.

4 Turn into an individual glass dish and chill before serving.

2.5 ml/½ tsp instant coffee granules

5 ml/1 tsp cocoa (unsweetened chocolate) powder

5 ml/1 tsp boiling water

10 ml/2 tsp artificial sweetener

1 egg white

45 ml/3 tbsp double (heavy) cream

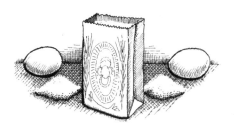

Serves 1

Carbohydrates: 2 g

Fresh lemon and lime sorbet

A cool, refreshing dessert that's perfect for rounding off any meal. You can't make one portion of this, so I've included it in several daily menus in this phase.

15 ml/1 tbsp powdered gelatine

175 ml/6 fl oz/³⁄₄ cup water

Finely grated zest and juice of 1 lime

Finely grated zest of 1 lemon

Juice of 4 lemons

Artificial sweetener, to taste

1 egg white

1 Mix the gelatine with 45 ml/3 tbsp of the water and leave to soften for 5 minutes. Either stand the bowl in a pan of hot water and stir until completely dissolved or heat briefly in the microwave – but do not boil.

2 Stir in the remaining water, the lime and lemon zests and juices.

3 Sweeten to taste with artificial sweetener – it should taste very sweet but still 'tangy'.

4 Pour the mixture into a freezer-proof container, cover and freeze for 2 hours or until firm around the edges.

5 Whisk thoroughly with a fork to break up the ice crystals. Whisk the egg white until stiff and fold in with a metal spoon. Re-cover and freeze for a further 1½ hours, then whisk thoroughly with a fork again. Cover and freeze until firm.

6 When ready to serve, transfer the sorbet to the fridge for 15 minutes beforehand, to soften slightly. Pop the rest back in the freezer as soon as possible.

Serves 6

Carbohydrates: 1 g per serving

Emmental with radishes and black pepper

Crisp, slightly peppery radishes are the ideal partners for the contrasting texture and slightly sweet, nutty flavour of Swiss cheese or any other of a similar texture.

1 Spear a cube of cheese and a radish on each of eight cocktail sticks (toothpicks).
2 Serve with a little ground black pepper to dip in.

25 g/1 oz Emmental (Swiss) cheese, cut into 8 cubes
8 radishes, trimmed
Freshly ground black pepper

Serves 1
Carbohydrates: 1 g

Mixed cheese platter with fresh fennel

The aniseed flavour of fennel and its cool crispness perfectly complement all kinds of cheese. I have suggested a mixture of hard, soft and blue cheeses but you can choose your favourites.

1 Arrange the cheeses on a platter.
2 Put the fennel to one side and season with pepper. Chill until ready to serve.

4 small wedges of cheese, such as Cheddar, Dolcelatte, Red Leicester and Camembert
¼ head of fennel, cut into small wedges
Freshly ground black pepper

Serves 1
Carbohydrates: 1 g

Smooth baked vanilla cream

A delicious, smooth, baked custard, this makes the perfect end to any meal. You can increase the quantity to serve the whole family but it will take longer to set in the oven.

75 ml/5 tbsp double (heavy) cream

30 ml/2 tbsp water

10 ml/ 2 tsp artificial sweetener

1 egg yolk

A few drops of vanilla essence (extract)

1 Whisk the cream with the water and sweetener. Whisk the egg yolk in thoroughly and then whisk in the vanilla essence.

2 Pour the mixture into a ramekin dish (custard cup) and stand it in a small baking tin (pan) or other ovenproof dish with enough boiling water to come halfway up the sides. Bake for about 30 minutes at 160°C/325°F/ gas 3/fan oven 145°C or until just set. Alternatively, stand the dish in a frying pan (skillet) with enough boiling water to come halfway up the sides, cover and simmer very gently for about 35 minutes until just set.

3 Serve warm or cold.

Serves 1

Carbohydrates: 2 g

St Clements jelly with crème fraîche

An ordinary jelly transformed into an elegant dessert. You can make a smaller quantity, but it's easier to make enough for four. As it has only a trace of carbohydrates, you can enjoy it anytime!

1 Dissolve the jelly crystals in the boiling water. Stir in the cold water and sharpen to taste with lemon juice.

2 Whisk in the crème fraîche until thoroughly blended, then pour into a serving dish, if using it all at once, or a plastic container with a lid. Chill until set. You can store it in the fridge for several days.

1 packet of sugar-free orange jelly crystals
150 ml/¼ pt/⅔ cup boiling water
300 ml/½ pt/1¼ cups cold water
25–30 ml/1–2 tbsp pure lemon juice
60 ml/4 tbsp crème fraîche

Serves 4
Carbohydrates:
Trace per serving

Chilled lime crème

This creamy dessert has a wonderfully tangy lime flavour but is equally delicious made with lemon if you wish to ring the changes. It makes a really refreshing pudding.

1 Mix the lime zest and juice in a small bowl with the crème fraîche.

2 Sweeten to taste with the artificial sweetener. Turn into a ramekin dish (custard cup) and chill until ready to serve.

Finely grated zest and juice of ½ lime
75 ml/5 tbsp crème fraîche
15 ml/1 tbsp artificial sweetener

Serves 1
Carbohydrates: 1 g

Creamy chocolate custard dessert

This velvety pudding is similar to the commercial chocolate desserts you can buy in the chiller cabinet at your favourite supermarket - but has far fewer carbohydrates.

5 ml/1 tsp cocoa (unsweetened chocolate) powder

90 ml/6 tbsp boiling water

30 ml/2 tbsp double (heavy) cream

1 egg

15 ml/1 tbsp artificial sweetener

1 Blend the cocoa with the boiling water in a small heavy-based saucepan.

2 Add the cream and whisk in the egg. Cook over a gentle heat, stirring all the time with a wooden spoon, until thickened. Do not allow to boil. Add the sweetener.

3 Spoon into a wine goblet and cover with clingfilm (plastic wrap) to prevent a skin forming. Leave to cool, then chill until ready to serve.

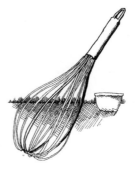

Serves 1

Carbohydrates: 1 g

Mediterranean-style coffee granita

A cool and refreshing way to round off a delicious meal. You can make as much of this as you like, but if you leave it until really hard, you'll have to crush it in a blender or food processor!

1 Mix the water with the coffee until dissolved, then add the artificial sweetener – it should taste very sweet.

2 Pour the mixture into a freezer-proof container and leave to cool. Freeze for about 1 hour until frozen around the edges. Whisk well with a fork to break up the ice crystals. Repeat the freezing and whisking twice more – it should take about 3 hours in all – until granular.

3 Spoon into a glass and serve.

150 ml/¼ pt/⅔ cup boiling water

10 ml/2 tsp instant coffee granules

15 ml/1 tbsp artificial sweetener

Serves 1
Carbohydrates: 1 g

Light frosted orange jelly snow

This is a simple way to transform an ordinary orange jelly into a light and luscious dessert. It uses the full packet of jelly but, as it's carb-free, you can eat as much as you like.

1 packet of orange sugar-free jelly (jello) crystals

150 ml/¼ pt/⅔ cup boiling water

300 ml/½ pt/1¼ cups cold water

1 egg, separated

1 Empty the jelly crystals into a bowl. Add the boiling water and stir until dissolved.

2 Stir in the cold water.

3 Whisk the egg yolk in another bowl and gradually whisk in the jelly. Chill until on the point of setting.

4 Whisk the egg white until stiff and fold into the mixture with a metal spoon. Chill again until set.

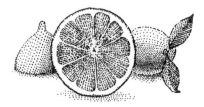

Serves 4

Carbohydrates: 0 g

Quick and easy lemon snow

It's not worth making this for one, but since you can enjoy it after any meal, it won't take long to finish it even if you are only preparing it for yourself.

1 Make up the jelly crystals according to the packet directions, using the lemon juice instead of 15 ml/1 tbsp of the water.

2 Chill until on the point of setting (when the mixture is the consistency of egg white).

3 Whisk the egg white until stiff, then fold it into the mixture using a metal spoon.

4 Turn into four glass dishes and chill until set.

1 packet of sugar-free jelly crystals

15 ml/1 tbsp lemon juice

1 egg white

Serves 4
Carbohydrates:
0 g per serving

Blue-cheese-stuffed cucumber

A soft, creamy blue cheese like Dolcelatte is ideal for making this cool and appetising savoury but you can substitute your favourite blue cheese if you prefer.

25 g/1 oz/¼ cup crumbled soft blue cheese

15 g/½ oz/1 tbsp softened butter

A pinch of grated nutmeg

5 cm/2 in piece of cucumber

1 Mash the cheese with the butter and nutmeg.

2 Cut the cucumber in half lengthways. Scoop out the seeds with a teaspoon and discard. Dry the cucumber with kitchen paper (paper towels).

3 Pack the cheese into the cucumber and chill until ready to serve.

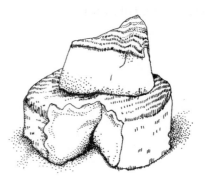

Serves 1

Carbohydrates: 2 g

Rich and creamy strawberry mousse layer

You wouldn't believe a packet jelly could make such a rich, creamy and fluffy mousse. It's not worth making less than this quantity but it will keep in the fridge or you can share it!

1 Add the jelly to the boiling water and stir until dissolved. Stir in the cold water and then the cream.

2 Whisk the egg white until stiff and fold in immediately. Pour into a glass dish or individual glasses. Chill until set. The mixture should separate into a fluffy layer with a smooth layer underneath.

Note: Since you don't need the egg yolk, poach it in a little water until hard, then store it in the fridge. Rub through a sieve to use as an attractive carb-free garnish for a salad or fish dish.

1 packet of strawberry sugar-free jelly (jello) crystals

150 ml/¼ pt/⅔ cup boiling water

300 ml/½ pt/1¼ cups cold water

4 tbsp single (light) cream

1 egg white

Serves 4
Carbohydrates:
1 g per serving

95

Melted Camembert with blackcurrant and celery

Warm, melting white cheese wedges, served with crisp celery and a drizzle of blackcurrant to offset the richness and complement the flavours.

2 wedges of Camembert

A little olive oil, for greasing

1 celery stick, cut into matchsticks

5 ml/1 tsp undiluted sugar-free real blackcurrant cordial

1 Put the Camembert on oiled foil on the grill (broiler) rack. Cook under a preheated grill for 1–2 minutes until beginning to melt.

2 Transfer to a warm plate with the celery. Quickly trickle the blackcurrant cordial over the cheese and serve straight away while the cheese is still runny.

Serves 1

Carbohydrates: 1 g

Blackcurrant fluff

This delicious recipe is my non-alcoholic version of Italian zabaglione. Try making it with other flavoured cordials too – but check their carbohydrate content before using them.

1 egg

15 ml/1 tbsp undiluted sugar-free real blackcurrant cordial

1 Break the egg into a bowl and whisk in the cordial.

2 Put the bowl over a pan of gently simmering water and whisk continuously until thick and fluffy. Spoon into a glass and serve.

Serves 1

Carbohydrates: Trace

Rhubarb fool with fresh ginger

Two ever-popular traditional flavours are blended together in this recipe to make the perfect fruit fool, rich and creamy but with just a hint of spice.

1 Put the rhubarb in a pan. Heat very gently until the juice runs, then cover the pan and cook over a gentle heat until really soft, stirring occasionally.

2 If there is still quite a lot of juice, boil rapidly to evaporate it, stirring all the time. Stir in the ginger and sweetener to taste. Remove from the heat and leave until cold.

3 Whip the cream until stiff. Fold in the cold rhubarb until just blended. Spoon into a glass and chill until ready to serve.

1 stick of rhubarb, cut into short lengths

1.5 ml/¼ tsp grated fresh root ginger

Artificial sweetener, to taste

45 ml/3 tbsp double (heavy) cream

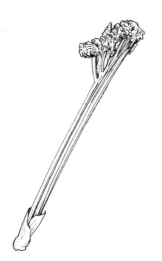

Serves 1
Carbohydrates: 2 g

Almond-flavoured jelly cream

When you are further along your path to weight loss, try serving this cool, smooth jelly with some fresh raspberries (an added 5 g carbs per portion) for an even more tempting dessert.

5 ml/1 tsp powdered gelatine

90 ml/6 tbsp water

60 ml/4 tbsp crème fraîche

A few drops of almond essence (extract)

Artificial sweetener, to taste

1 Mix the gelatine with 15 ml/1 tbsp of the water in a small bowl. Leave to soften for 5 minutes.

2 Stand the bowl in a pan of gently simmering water and stir until completely dissolved (the quantity is not large enough to use the microwave).

3 Stir in the remaining cold water, then whisk in 45 ml/3 tbsp of the crème fraîche. Add almond essence and sweetener to taste.

4 Pour into a small glass dish and chill until set. Top with the remaining crème fraîche before serving.

Serves 1
Carbohydrates: 2 g

Phase 2: Gradual Weight Loss

In Phase 2, you are now aiming to lose 500 g–1 kg/1–2 lb per week in a gradual, continuing process. You must eat more carbs than you were doing in the induction phase or you may become ill, but if you increase your intake of carbs too quickly, you may not lose any more weight or you may even start to put weight on again. Clearly, it is important to get this phase right, so you must monitor both your carbohydrate intake and your weight very carefully.

In the first week of Phase 2, you increase your daily carbohydrate count by 5 g, to 25 g per day, using the menus from Phase 1 and adding in 'top-ups' from a list of allowed foods. A full explanation of how to do this is given later in the chapter (see Phase 2, Week 1, starting on page 100). You should continue this at this level for one week.

If you are still losing weight, you can move on to Week 2, increasing the daily carb intake by 10 g (to 35 g per day). Again, there are full details of how to do this (see Phase 2, Week 2, starting on page 103). Continue in this way, increasing your daily carbohydrate intake by 10 g each week, using the lists of recommended foods and the menus in this chapter, making sure that you are still losing weight. If you find 10 g per week is too drastic a leap, try 5 g increments.

This phase of the diet can last as long as necessary. The important thing is to gradually increase your carbohydrates, while still losing weight, until you have lost nearly all the weight you need. The time it takes and the quantity of carbohydrates will differ from person to person.

As in Phase 1, this chapter provides you with lists of foods that you can eat, and also a selection of recipes that you can use from the fourth week of your diet (Phase 2, Week 2). Each of the recipes gives you all the information you need to tailor it to suit your own tastes and you will soon learn to manage your carbohydrates perfectly. You can mix and match meals as you like, to add up to the daily carbohydrate count you need. As before, make sure you eat all the fruit and vegetables suggested, or exchange them for ones with the same carbohydrate count. You can, of course, use the recipes from Phase 1, but increase the amount of vegetables already allowed, to increase your carbohydrates allowance.

Drinks

Now you may have a dash of fortified unsweetened soya milk in your tea or coffee instead of cream, if you prefer. You may also have a glass or two of wine (preferably red), or a spirit with a calorie-free mixer, but don't drink to excess (remember, your body will burn the alcohol **before** fat for energy). Avoid sweet drinks, both alcoholic and non-alcoholic, and only have pure fruit juices where part of the meal plan. Drink plenty of water.

Watch points
LOW FIBRE

The lack of fibre on a low-carbohydrate diet can cause problems with the body's digestive system. As stressed already, it is very important that you drink plenty of water, eat lots of nuts and seeds and as many fruit and vegetables as you are allowed and take plenty of exercise. If you find that you do suffer from constipation, try sprinkling flax meal or seeds on your food (follow the directions on the packet). Alternatively, an extra tablespoon of olive oil a day (maybe on your salad) can help. If not, you can buy natural health preparations from your health food shop, which should help.

Phase 2, Week 1

This is the third week of your diet and you now are going to increase your daily carbohydrate counts by 5 g. The easiest way to do this is to use the menus from Phase 1 (see pages 22–7) and add in any one quantity of the nuts, seeds or fruits given in the list on page 101. Alternatively, you can add in two half portions: for example, on Day 1 of the diet (see page 23), you could sprinkle your Caesar Salad for lunch with 2½ tbsp sunflower seeds and have 40 g/1½ oz/generous heaped tbsp sliced strawberries with the jelly (jello) for pudding – easy!

You must continue to have each complete day's menus as you did in Phase 1. Remember to eat **everything** on the menu or substitute items of equal carbohydrate value. Continue to monitor your weight as before.

ADDITIONS – 5 G
Nuts and seeds
Each measured amount here contains 5 g of carbohydrate. You can also choose your 5 g 'top-ups' from this list or from the Phase 1 lists starting on page 20. If you use foods from the earlier list, make sure you have enough to give you 5 g of carbohydrate.

- 5 tbsp (35 g/1¼ oz/good ¼ cup) of cashew nuts
- 5 tbsp (35 g/1¼ oz/good ¼ cup) of pumpkin or sunflower or sesame seeds
- 7 tbsp (45 g/1¾ oz/scant ½ cup) of peanuts
- 10 tbsp (65 g/2½ oz/good ½ cup) of macadamias, mixed nuts, pecans or pistachios
- 20 tbsp (150 g/5 oz/1¼ cups) brazils, hazelnuts (filberts), pine nuts or walnuts

Where the quantities of nuts are large, it is probably best to split half a portion with half a portion of one of the fruits in the list on the next page.

If you want to eat all of one type of nut, you may not fancy munching your way through that many, so a good way of enjoying them is to make a nut butter or cream. For nut butter, purée them in a blender or food processor, adding a dash of sunflower or nut oil to form a paste, stopping and scraping down the sides as necessary. Season with a tiny pinch of salt, if necessary, then spread it in celery for a delicious snack. For nut cream, purée the nuts in a blender or food processor with a little water (about 60 ml/4 tbsp per 50 g/2 oz/½ cup nuts) to form a soft dropping consistency. Sweeten with a little artificial sweetener. Chill until ready to serve on any of the desserts in the diet plan or with sugar-free jelly (jello) for a snack.

Fruits

Each of the measured portions given here contains 5 g of carbohydrates.

- 100 g/4 oz/3 heaped tbsp raspberries or blackberries
- 75 g/3 oz/2½ heaped tbsp sliced strawberries
- 1 fresh fig
- 1 guava
- 12 cherries
- 10 physalis
- 5 fresh lychees

Vegetables

Alternatively, on some days, you can add more vegetables from the list on page 20. Choose from the following:

- An average serving (50 g/2 oz) of mixed salad
- A large (100 g/4 oz) green salad
- An average portion (100 g/4 oz) of cooked carrots, kohlrabi or green (French) beans
- A large green (bell) pepper
- A small yellow or orange pepper or ½ medium red pepper

For variety, you could try a combination of vegetables, such as a portion of broccoli and a portion of mangetout; a portion of leeks and a portion of runner beans; a portion of cabbage and a portion of courgettes (zucchini).

Phase 2, Week 2 onwards

You now increase your daily intake of carbohydrates to 35 g for a week. Each day, select a breakfast, a lunch and a dinner from the menus and recipes in this section. You will also find suggestions for additional carbohydrates you can add after that to increase the amount per week by 5 or 10 g per day. If you try adding an extra 10 g carbohydrate per day and find, after a week, you are beginning to gain weight again, cut the carbohydrates by 5 g. An easy way to cut, if you have to, is to leave out your dessert after dinner!

MORE FOODS YOU ARE ALLOWED

You can now have portions of the following as well as all the previously allowed foods and additions.

* 4 tbsp = 25 g/1 oz/¼ cup
** 1 tbsp = 7.5 g/¼ oz
*** 3 heaped tbsp = 100 g/4 oz

Nuts and seeds

Those in this list are very low in carbohydrates but high in fibre.

Item	Quantity	Carb content
Almonds	4 tbsp*	2 g
Brazils	4 tbsp*	1 g
Cashews	4 tbsp*	4 g
Coconut, desiccated	1 tbsp**	1 g
Fennel seeds	1 tbsp**	trace
Hazelnuts (filberts)	4 tbsp*	1 g
Macadamias	4 tbsp*	2 g
Mixed nuts	4 tbsp*	2 g
Peanuts	4 tbsp*	3 g
Pecans	4 tbsp*	2 g
Pine nuts	4 tbsp*	1 g
Pistachios	4 tbsp*	2 g
Pumpkin seeds	1 tbsp**	1 g
Sesame seeds	1 tbsp**	trace
Sunflower seeds	1 tbsp**	1 g
Walnuts	4 tbsp*	1 g

Fruits

Item	Quantity	Carb content
Apricot, dried	1	3 g
Apricot, fresh	1	4 g
Blackberries	3 heaped tbsp***	5 g
Blackcurrants	3 heaped tbsp***	7 g
Cherries	12	5 g
Clementine	1	6 g
Damson	1	1 g
Date, fresh	1	8 g
Fig, fresh	1	5 g
Guava	1	5 g
Gooseberries	3 heaped tbsp***	2 g
Grapefruit	½	6 g
Greengage	1	2 g
Kumquat	1	3 g
Lychee	1	1 g
Mandarin orange	1	7 g
Passion fruit	1	4 g
Persimmon	1	8 g
Physalis	1	trace
Plum	1 small	2 g
Plum	1 large	7 g
Prune	1	3 g
Raspberries	3 heaped tbsp***	5 g
Satsuma	1	5 g
Starfruit	1	7 g
Strawberries, sliced	3 heaped tbsp***	6 g

Other foods

For even more variety, you can substitute the following for other foods with a similar carbohydrate allowance.

Item	Quantity	Carb content
Wild rice, uncooked	50 g/2 oz/¼ cup	6 g

(Do not confuse this with wild rice mix, which is half long-grain white rice and so has a much higher carb content.)

Sauerkraut	3 heaped tbsp***	5 g
Soya beans (soaked and cooked)	3 heaped tbsp***	5 g
Full-fat soya flour	4 tbsp*	6 g

(This is much lower in carbs than wheat or other grain flours, so good for baking.)

Fortified unsweetened soya milk	300 ml/½ pt/1¼ cups	2 g
Greek-style strained yoghurt made with cows' milk	100 ml/3½ fl oz/ scant ½ cup	4 g
Crispbread, rye	1 slice	6 g
Crispbread, starch-reduced	1 slice	3 g
Crispbread, wheat	1 slice	7 g
Crisp rice cakes	1	7 g

ADDITIONS – 10 G

As you progress through Phase 2, you will be gradually increasing your carbohydrates (see page 99). When you want to add 10 g of carbohydrates, choose from any of these snacks, or have any of the fruits, nuts and seeds that add up to 10 g carbohydrates from the lists given earlier.

10 g snacks

- A small handful (15 g/½ oz) of dried banana slices

- A small handful (15 g/½ oz) of raisins or sultanas

- A handful (25 g/1 oz) of peanuts and raisins

- 1 dried date

- 1 small kiwi fruit

- 1 tumbler (250 ml/8 fl oz) pure apple juice

- 1 cream cracker/water biscuit with cheese and 5 ml/1 tsp sweet pickle or chutney

- 1 taco shell with grated cheese, 1 sliced tomato, a handful of shredded lettuce and 5 slices of cucumber

- 1 starch-reduced bread roll, buttered, if liked

- 1 rollmop, sliced, on 1 buttered starch-reduced crispbread

- 10 sticks of cheese and pineapple

10 g side dishes

- 100 g/4 oz/3 heaped tbsp cooked fresh shelled or frozen peas

- 1 medium cooked beetroot (red beet), with or without vinegar

- 100 g/4 oz/3 heaped tbsp cooked soya beans and 1 diced green (bell) pepper, in mayonnaise or oil and vinegar dressing, flavoured with snipped chives

Phase 2, Week 4 onwards

After two weeks, if you are still losing weight, you can add one of these to any of the basic 35 g menus
(1 breakfast, 1 lunch and 1 dinner). This is of course **instead of,** not as well as, any of the 5 g or 10 g additions already mentioned. If you find they are too much and you start to gain weight again, stop eating them immediately and go back to the 10 g additions. (You should be able to include them as 'treats' when you get to Phase 3.)

ADDITIONS – 11–15 G

- 100 g/4 oz/3 heaped tbsp cooked, frozen broad (fava) beans
- 100 g/4 oz/3 heaped tbsp Jerusalem artichokes, mashed or puréed with butter or cream
- 100 g/4 oz/3 heaped tbsp parsnips, mashed, with butter, if liked
- 100 g/4 oz/3 heaped tbsp ratatouille
- 1 small or ½ large corn-on-the-cob, with melted butter, if liked
- 1 medium apple
- 1 medium peach
- 1 medium nectarine
- 1 medium pear
- 1 medium orange
- 1 slice of fresh pineapple
- 1 medium pomegranate
- ½ medium mango

- ½ medium papaya
- 1 large wedge of honeydew or water melon or ½ small round melon e.g. cantaloupe
- 100 g/4 oz/3 heaped tbsp canned fruit, in natural juice
- 100 g/4 oz grapes
- 125 ml/4½ oz/1 small pot of Greek-style yoghurt, with honey
- 300 ml/½ pt/1¼ cups cows' milk

Breakfasts

Each of these breakfasts is specially designed to give you an allowance of 10 g of carbohydrates. You may swap items provided that your total adds up to 10 g for your complete breakfast. I suggest you always have a fruit option as it helps provide your vitamin and mineral content for the day to keep you fit and well.

Choose from any of the following combinations:

1 small glass (120 ml/4 fl oz) pure orange juice	7 g carb
1 or 2 eggs, fried (sautéed) or poached, and	
2 rashers (slices) of bacon, fried or grilled (broiled)	0 g carb
1 crisp Italian breadstick	3 g carb
½ grapefruit, with artificial sweetener, if liked	6 g carb
2 Creamy Scrambled Eggs (see page 30) and	
1 tomato, grilled (broiled)	2 g carb
on 1 slice of Low-carbohydrate Soya Bread	
(see page 113), toasted and buttered	2 g carb
1 small glass (120 ml/4 fl oz) tomato juice	3 g carb
Slices of salami and a selection of cheeses	0 g carb
1 wheat crispbread or a crisp rice cake, buttered	7 g carb
1 small glass (120 ml/4 fl oz) pure apple juice	5 g carb
2–3 rashers (slices) of bacon, fried (sautéed)	
or grilled (broiled), with stewed or fried mushrooms	
and a dash of Worcestershire sauce	1 g carb
1 slice of Low-carbohydrate Soya Bread	
(see page 113), toasted, with 1 tbsp peanut butter	4 g carb

1 clementine	6 g carb
2 boiled eggs	0 g carb
2 slices of Low-carbohydrate Soya Bread	
(see page 113), toasted and buttered	4 g carb
¼ medium cantaloupe, galia or ogen melon	7 g carb
Plain, cheese or mushroom omelette, made with	
2 eggs (see page 39 for basic method)	0 g carb
1 crisp Italian breadstick	3 g carb
½ grapefruit, with artificial sweetener, if liked	6 g carb
1 kipper, grilled (broiled) or poached	0 g carb
2 slices of Low-carbohydrate Soya Bread	
(see page 113), buttered	4 g carb
1 small tub (125 g/4½ oz) of cottage cheese	
with pineapple	3 g carb
1 tbsp pumpkin seeds	1 g carb
2 tbsp chopped hazelnuts (filberts)	1 g carb
3 heaped tbsp fresh or thawed frozen raspberries	
with artificial sweetener, if liked	5 g carb
1 small glass (120 ml/4 fl oz) pure apple juice	5 g carb
1 thick pure pork sausage, grilled (broiled) or	
fried (sautéed)	4 g carb
1 or 2 eggs, poached or fried	0 g carb
½ tomato, grilled	1 g carb
100 ml/3½ fl oz/scant ½ cup Greek-style strained	
yoghurt, made with cow's milk, with artificial	
sweetener, if liked	4 g carb
1 passion fruit	4 g carb
1 tbsp chopped brazils	trace carb
1 slice of Low-carbohydrate Soya Bread	
(see page 113), buttered, with Marmite	
or other yeast extract	2 g carb

Lunches

Your lunch should contain 10 g of carbohydrate in all, so that's exactly what all these combinations contain.

All the desserts contain 3 g and the rest of the lunch (which may include a soup and salad, to be eaten as part of the same meal) contains 7 g in all. Your lunch **must** include a dessert or savoury as well as the rest of the meal but you can mix and match them if you wish.

Clear Mixed Winter Vegetable Soup (see page 114)
Cheese-stuffed Eggs with Mixed Green Salad (see page 115)
Creamy Fresh Gooseberry Ripple (see page 156)

Tuna Mornay with Roasted Peanuts (see page 116)
Sliced Tomato and Fresh Chive Salad (see page 117)
Raspberry Crush Cream (see page 157)

Bagna Cauda with Vegetable Dippers (see page 118)
Selection of cheeses with 1 Italian bread stick

Quiche Lorraine with Soya and Celeriac Pastry (see page 120)
   with Rocket Salad (see page 121)
Citrus Jelly with Fresh Clementines (see page 159)

Fresh Sherried Chicken Broth with Herbs (see page 119)
Spicy Ham and Coleslaw Rolls (see page 112)
Chocolate Cheese with Walnuts (see page 158)

Salmon Mousse with Artichoke and Watercress (see page 125)
Light and Lacy Soya Crêpes with Lemon (see page 163)

Smoked Mackerel Pâté with Cucumber Boats (see page 122)
   with 1 crisp Italian breadstick
Devils and Angels on Horseback (see page 157)

Guacamole with Parmesan Wafers and Chicory (see page 123)
Creamy Yoghurt with Hazelnuts (see page 162)

Italian Delicatessen Meat and Cheese Platter (see page 124)
Coffee Honeycomb Mould with Pecans (see page 161)

Spiced Spanish Omelette with Pepper and Onion (see page 126)
Creamy Mousse with Fresh Strawberries (see page 160)

Dinners

Each dinner menu contains 15 g of carbohydrates.

Now you can really treat yourself! You should have a dessert as well as a main course – all the main courses are 10 g of carbohydrates, all the desserts are worth 5 g of carbohydrates, so you can swap them round as you fancy. You will also find a selection of no-carbohydrate starters, so, if you're celebrating or entertaining, you can have three courses with no extra carbohydrates. If you're serving someone who isn't on the regime, you can offer French bread or rolls.

I've made up a number of suggested menus, to get your taste buds working, but you can select whichever combinations you like. Remember, the starters are non-carbohydrate so you can eat them or not, as you wish – I suggest you have them for high days and holidays only! All recipes serve four people, but can easily be multiplied to six or cut down to one or two as necessary.

Parma Ham with Marinated Olives (see page 127)
Poussins with Pesto and Italian Roasted Vegetables
   (see page 154)
Apricot Zabaglione with a Saffron Bun (see page 168)

Seafood and Wild Rocket Salad (see page 131)
Chicken in Red Wine with Mangetout and Baby Corn
   (see page 140)
Mandarin Orange Cheese Sherbet (see page 167)

Watercress Roulade with Cream Cheese and Chives
   (see page 128)
Mushroom-topped Pork Chops with Red Cabbage
   (see page 142)
Whisky Lemon Syllabub with Coconut Dusting (see page 176)

Individual Baked Eggs with Pancetta (see page 130)
Warm Duck Breast Salad with Raspberries (see page 146)
Low-carbohydrate Italian Tiramisu (see page 175)

Carpacchio of Beef with Crushed Black Pepper (see page 133)
Poached Salmon with Baby Vegetables (see page 138)
Apricot and Persimmon Melba (see page 172)

Sesame-fried Camembert on Watercress (see page 132)
Thai Prawn and Cucumber Curry with Wild Rice
   (see page 150)
Hazelnut Cream with Raspberry Coulis (see page 166)

Smoked Salmon with Prawns and Lemon (see page 129)
Steak with Grainy Mustard Jus and Beetroot Chips
   (see page 148)
Potted Stilton with Red Wine and Fennel (see page 171)

Potted Prawns with Sweet Spices (see page 136)
Nutty Lamb Chops with Fresh Mint Jelly (see page 144)
Avocado Whip with a Dash of Lime (see page 174)

Chilli-spiced Scallops with Bacon (see page 135)
Turkey, Ham and Cheese Rolls with Tomato Coulis,
   (see page 152)
Strawberry and Greek Yoghurt Sesame Brûlée (see page 165)

King Prawns in Olive Oil and Garlic Butter (see page 134)
Chicken and Vegetable Stir-fry (see page 139)
Fresh Lychees with Ripe French Brie (see page 164)

Breakfast and Lunch Recipes

This selection of recipes will really start to broaden your scope of exciting eating. The bread recipe on page 113 makes an excellent breakfast loaf. Enjoy it sliced fresh or toasted with butter. It can also be used for breadcrumbs to coat meat, fish or chicken before frying and even for desserts. The other breakfast suggestions given in the menus on pages 107–8 don't need recipes, so the remainder of the recipes in this section are for lunchtime.

All the lunch recipes are exciting, tasty and nutritious. As I've said before, where you've been given a soup and a salad, you must eat both. The combination will add up to 7 g of carbohydrates and then you must have your pudding, too, which contains 3 g of carbohydrates. If you choose to swap items, make sure you have the same total number of carbohydrates for the meal.

Spicy ham and coleslaw rolls

Rolls of tender ham wrapped round crisp, creamy coleslaw, lifted with a dash of Tabasco to give it a zing. Watch out for low-fat coleslaws, as they are likely to be higher in carbohydrates.

4 slices of ham

100 g/4 oz ready-made coleslaw

Tabasco sauce

5 slices of cucumber

Serves 1
Carbohydrates: 7 g

1 Lay the slices of ham on a board. Spoon the coleslaw across each slice towards one end.

2 Add a few drops of Tabasco to each pile of coleslaw. Roll up and transfer to a plate.

3 Serve garnished with the cucumber slices.

Low-carbohydrate soya bread

This is a light and tasty bread, the ideal choice for breakfast, lunch or dinner. At only 2 g carbohydrates per slice, you can enjoy it in place of wheat bread any time.

1 Sift the soya flour, baking powder and salt together.

2 Beat the egg yolks with the butter and crème fraîche until well blended.

3 Beat in the flour mixture.

4 Whisk the egg whites until stiff. Beat 30 ml/2 tbsp into the soya flour mixture to slacken it, then fold in the remainder with a metal spoon.

5 Turn into a greased 450 g/1 lb loaf tin (pan), base-lined with non-stick baking parchment, and bake in a preheated oven at 180°C/350°F/ gas 4/fan oven 160°C for about 40 minutes or until risen, golden and firm to the touch.

6 Turn out on a wire rack to cool, then store in a polythene bag in the fridge for up to 3 days, or slice and freeze.

50 g/2 oz/½ cup full-fat soya flour

15 ml/1 tbsp baking powder

A good pinch of salt

4 eggs, separated

40 g/1½ oz/3 tbsp butter, melted

45 ml/3 tbsp crème fraîche

Makes 1 loaf (10 slices)
Carbohydrates: 2 g per slice

Clear mixed winter vegetable soup

This is a brilliant way to get a good portion of your five-a-day vegetables in one bowl! It's filling, colourful, very nutritious – and exceptionally tasty into the bargain.

1 carrot, coarsely grated

1 turnip, coarsely grated

¼ head of celeriac (celery root), coarsely grated

1 litre/1¾ pts/4¼ cups vegetable stock, made with 1½ stock cubes

2.5 ml/½ tsp Marmite or other yeast extract

1 bay leaf

Freshly ground black pepper

1 Put all the ingredients in a saucepan. Bring to the boil, reduce the heat, part-cover and simmer for 10 minutes.

2 Remove the bay leaf and season with more pepper, if necessary. Ladle into warm bowls to serve.

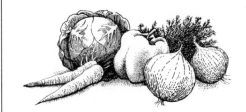

Serves 4

Carbohydrates: 4 g per serving

Cheese-stuffed eggs with mixed green salad

Hard-boiled egg yolk blended with creamy blue cheese, mayonnaise and freshly ground black pepper, then piled back into the whites and served on a bed of salad.

1 Shell the egg and cut in half. Scoop out the yolk into a bowl.

2 Mash well with the cheese and mayonnaise, then season with pepper to taste.

3 Pile the cheese mixture back into the hollows of the egg white halves.

4 Arrange the salad leaves, pepper and cucumber on a plate. Top with the stuffed eggs and add a cluster of cress between the egg halves.

1 egg, hard-boiled (hard-cooked)

25 g/1 oz soft blue cheese

15 ml/1 tbsp mayonnaise

Freshly ground black pepper

A good handful of mixed salad leaves

¼ green (bell) pepper, thinly sliced

5 slices of cucumber

A good handful of salad cress

Serves 1
Carbohydrates: 3 g

Tuna mornay with roasted peanuts

A sizzling blend of tuna, peanuts and cheese. Smaller cans of tuna are much more expensive, so if eating alone, have the remainder cold or reheated in the microwave the next day.

1 x 185 g/6½ oz/small can of tuna, drained

50 g/2 oz/½ cup roasted peanuts

75 ml/5 tbsp crème fraîche

75 ml/5 tbsp water

1 egg, beaten

Freshly ground black pepper

2.5 ml/½ tsp dried mixed herbs

50 g/2 oz/½ cup grated Cheddar cheese

15 ml/1 tbsp chopped fresh parsley

Serve with:

A Sliced Tomato and Fresh Chive Salad (see page 117)

1 Empty the tuna into a shallow ovenproof dish. Mix in the nuts.

2 Beat the crème fraîche, water and egg together with some black pepper and the dried mixed herbs. Spoon it over the tuna and peanuts.

3 Sprinkle the cheese liberally over the surface.

4 Bake in a preheated oven at 190°C/375°F/gas 5/fan oven 170°C for about 30 minutes until just set, golden and bubbling.

5 Sprinkle with the chopped parsley and serve hot with a Sliced Tomato and Fresh Chive Salad.

Serves 2

Carbohydrates: 7 g per serving (including 4 g for the Tomato and Chive Salad)

Sliced tomato and fresh chive salad

A colourful, refreshing blend of ingredients makes this an ideal accompaniment to any meat, poultry or fish dishes, especially my Tuna Mornay with Roasted Peanuts.

1 Arrange the tomatoes in a single layer in two shallow dishes. Sprinkle liberally with the chives.

2 Whisk the oil, vinegar and seasonings together and drizzle over the salad. Leave to stand for about 30 minutes before serving, to allow the flavours to develop, if time allows.

4 tomatoes, sliced

30 ml/2 tbsp snipped fresh chives

15 ml/1 tbsp olive oil

5 ml/1 tsp red wine vinegar

A pinch of artificial sweetener

Salt and freshly ground black pepper

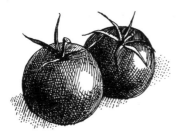

Serves 2

Carbohydrates: 4 g per serving

Bagna cauda
with vegetable dippers

A Mediterranean speciality: anchovies, olive oil, garlic and butter blended to an unctuous dip, served with crisp vegetables. It's too much for one, so store the rest in the fridge and reheat it.

1 head of chicory
(Belgian endive)

1 green (bell) pepper,
cut into strips

2 small carrots, cut
into short sticks

4 celery sticks, cut into
short sticks

For the dip:

1 x 50 g/2 oz/small can
of anchovies

75 ml/5 tbsp olive oil

1 garlic clove, crushed

25 g/1 oz/2 tbsp
unsalted (sweet)
butter

1 Cut a cone-shaped core out of the base of the chicory, then separate the head into leaves. Chill all the prepared vegetables until ready to serve.

2 Drain the oil from the anchovies into a saucepan. Add the olive oil and garlic. Chop the fish finely and add to the pan.

3 Heat, stirring, until gently simmering and the fish 'melts' into the oil.

4 Beat in the butter, a little at a time, until glistening.

5 Pour the mixture into two small bowls and place on plates with the vegetable 'dippers' around.

6 Serve while still hot.

Serves 2

Carbohydrates:
6 g per serving

Fresh sherried chicken broth with herbs

You can also make this delicious clear soup with a cooked chicken carcass. If you only need one serving, it can be stored in the fridge for several days, or frozen in individual portions.

1 Put all the ingredients except the sherry in a saucepan. Bring to the boil and skim the surface.

2 Reduce the heat, cover and simmer very gently for 1½ hours.

3 Strain the stock and return it to the rinsed-out saucepan.

4 When cool enough to handle, carefully pick all the meat off the bones, discarding the skin. Chop the flesh and return it to the pan. Stir in the sherry. Taste and re-season, if necessary.

5 Reheat and serve hot.

1 chicken leg portion

1 onion, washed and quartered, but not peeled

1 celery stick, chopped

1 bouquet garni sachet

1 chicken stock cube

1 litre/1¾ pts/4¼ cups water

Salt and freshly ground black pepper

45 ml/3 tbsp dry sherry

Serves 4
Carbohydrates:
Trace per serving

Quiche Lorraine
with soya and celeriac pastry

The perfect alternative to high-carb pastry, this is really low in carbs with a lovely nutty flavour. You could make a larger quantity and freeze the remainder or store it in the fridge for three days.

100 g/4 oz/¼ peeled celeriac (celery root), cut into small chunks

85 g/3½ oz/scant 1 cup full-fat soya flour

45 ml/3 tbsp olive oil

Salt

About 15 ml/1 tbsp cold water

For the filling:

4 rashers (slices) of streaky bacon, rinded and diced

4 spring onions (scallions), chopped

2.5 ml/½ tsp dried mixed herbs

75 g/3 oz/¾ cup grated Cheddar cheese

2 eggs

300 ml/½ pt/1¼ cups unsweetened enriched soya milk

Freshly ground black pepper

Serves 4

Carbohydrates: 7 g per serving

1 Boil the celeriac in water for 10 minutes until tender. Drain and mash well.

2 Mix in the flour, oil and a pinch of salt, then add just enough water to form a soft but not sticky dough. Wrap in clingfilm (plastic wrap) and chill for at least 30 minutes.

3 Roll out the pastry (paste) thinly and use to line an 20 cm/8 in flan dish (pie pan) on a baking (cookie) sheet. Prick the base with a fork and line with foil.

4 Bake in a preheated oven at 200°C/ 400°F/gas 6/fan oven 180°C for 10 minutes. Remove the foil and return to the oven for 5 minutes to dry out.

5 Meanwhile, dry-fry the bacon with the onions in a frying pan (skillet), stirring, until the bacon is almost cooked and the onions have softened.

6 Tip the mixture into the cooked flan case (pie shell) and sprinkle with the herbs and cheese.

7 Beat the eggs with the milk and season with salt and pepper. Pour into the flan. Bake in the oven at 190°C/375°F/gas 5/fan oven 170°C for about 30 minutes until golden and set.

8 Serve warm or cold.

Rocket salad with sesame seeds

A blend of peppery rocket, fragrant coriander and sweet salad cress, dressed with sesame seeds fried in olive oil until lightly golden and blended with vinegar and seasonings.

1 Heat the oil in a frying pan (skillet). Add the sesame seeds and fry (sauté) until lightly golden, then remove from the heat immediately and leave to cool.

2 Mix the rocket, coriander and cress together in a salad bowl.

3 Mix the vinegar into the sesame seeds and oil and season to taste with salt, pepper and sweetener. Spoon over the salad and toss.

15 ml/1 tbsp olive oil

10 ml/2 tsp sesame seeds

A good handful of rocket

A sprig of fresh coriander (cilantro), torn into small pieces

A good handful of salad cress

5 ml/1 tsp red wine vinegar

Salt and freshly ground black pepper

A pinch of artificial sweetener

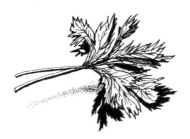

Serves 1

Carbohydrates: Trace

Smoked mackerel pâté with cucumber boats

Smoked mackerel, blended with cream cheese, pepper and butter, packed into chunks of cucumber. If eating alone, store any leftover pâté in the fridge or freezer. Try it with no-carb chicory.

1 smoked mackerel fillet, about 150 g/ 5 oz

25 g/1 oz/2 tbsp butter

25 g/1 oz/2 tbsp cream cheese

5–10 ml/1–2 tsp lemon juice

Freshly ground black pepper

2 x 10 cm/4 in pieces of cucumber

2 crisp Italian breadsticks

1 Remove the skin from the mackerel and put the fish in a blender or food processor with the butter and cheese. Run the machine until the mixture is smooth, stopping and scraping down the sides as necessary.

2 Season the pâté with lemon juice and a little pepper to taste.

3 Cut the cucumber pieces in half lengthways and scoop out the seeds. Pile the pâté into the cucumber 'boats' and serve each portion with one crisp breadstick.

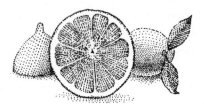

Serves 2

Carbohydrates: 7 g per serving

Guacamole with Parmesan wafers and chicory

This dip is made with avocado mashed with olive oil and a hint of onion, sharpened with lemon juice, Worcestershire and Tabasco sauces, then lightly mixed with tomato and cucumber.

1 Make the wafers. Oil a baking (cookie) sheet. Put 12 spoonfuls of Parmesan cheese in small piles a little apart on the sheet and flatten with a fork. Bake in a preheated oven at 200°C/400°F/gas 6/fan oven 180°C for 10 minutes until melted. Remove from the oven and leave to cool and become crisp. Store in an airtight container – they'll keep for days.

2 Make the guacamole. Halve the avocado, remove the stone (pit) and scoop the flesh out into a bowl. Mash well with a fork or balloon whisk.

3 Whisk in the lemon juice, then whisk in the oil a few drops at a time until thick and creamy.

4 Flavour with the onion, Tabasco and Worcestershire sauces and a little salt and pepper. Sharpen with more lemon juice, if liked.

5 Stir in the tomato and cucumber. Spoon into a small pot and put it on a plate.

6 Cut a cone-shaped core out of the base of the chicory, then separate it into leaves. Arrange around the guacamole and serve with as many Parmesan wafers as you like (0 carbs!).

For the Parmesan wafers:
100 g/4 oz/1 cup freshly grated Parmesan cheese

For the guacamole:
1 ripe avocado
A squeeze of lemon juice
30 ml/2 tbsp olive oil, plus extra for greasing
1.5 ml/'/₄ tsp grated onion
A few drops each of Tabasco and Worcestershire sauce
Salt and freshly ground black pepper
1 tomato, finely chopped
2.5 cm/1 in piece of cucumber, chopped
1 head of chicory (Belgian endive)

Serves 1
Carbohydrates: 7 g (including 0 g per wafer)

Italian delicatessen meat and cheese platter

A selection of continental meats, beautifully laid out with cool Mozzarella, peppery rocket and juicy tomato, drizzled with olive oil and a dash of balsamic vinegar - so simple but so delicious.

2 slices each of Parma ham, bresaola, mortadella, Milano salami and speck

1 x 100 g/4 oz/small fresh Mozzarella cheese, sliced

A good handful of rocket

1 plum tomato, sliced

15 ml/1 tbsp olive oil

5 ml/1 tsp balsamic vinegar

Freshly ground black pepper

1 Arrange the meats attractively on a large platter.

2 Tuck the cheese in between the meat slices.

3 Put a pile of rocket in the centre and arrange the tomato slices attractively around.

4 Drizzle the rocket and tomato with the oil and vinegar and add a good grinding of black pepper all over.

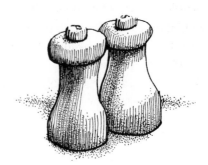

Serves 1
Carbohydrates: 7 g

Salmon mousse with artichoke and watercress

This delicately flavoured mousse tastes as good as any made with fresh salmon! If eating alone, use only half the salad and store the remaining mousse in the fridge for another day.

1 Drain off the liquor from the fish into a small bowl. Add the gelatine and leave to soften for 5 minutes. Stand the bowl in a pan of gently simmering water and stir until dissolved.

2 Beat in the egg yolk and continue to stir, with the bowl still in the hot water, until slightly thickened. Remove from the pan.

3 Remove the skin and bones from the fish.

4 Beat the fish into the yolk mixture. Season to taste with salt, pepper and lemon juice.

5 Whisk the egg white until stiff.

6 Fold the mayonnaise into the fish and then the egg white, using a metal spoon. Chill until set.

7 Arrange the salad stuffs on two plates. Spoon the mousse to one side and garnish with wedges of lemon. Serve each portion with a breadstick.

1 x 200 g/7 oz/small can of red salmon

10 ml/2 tsp powdered gelatine

1 egg, separated

90 ml/6 tbsp mayonnaise

Salt and freshly ground black pepper

A squeeze of lemon juice

2 handfuls of shredded lettuce

10 slices of cucumber

2 handfuls of watercress

2 artichoke hearts, quartered

30 ml/2 tbsp sunflower seeds

Wedges of lemon, for garnishing

Serve with:

2 Italian breadsticks

Serves 2

Carbohydrates: 7 g per serving (including 0 g for the mousse)

Spiced Spanish omelette with pepper and onion

A delicious version of a classic favourite: green pepper, onion and an artichoke heart cooked in a glorious golden omelette, judiciously spiced with chilli flakes. It's equally good hot or cold.

15 ml/1 tbsp olive oil

½ green (bell) pepper, thinly sliced

1 small onion, thinly sliced

3 eggs

30 ml/2 tbsp water

Salt and freshly ground black pepper

1 artichoke heart, sliced

1.5 ml/¼ tsp dried oregano

A good pinch of dried chilli flakes

A sprig of fresh parsley

1 Heat the oil in an omelette pan. Add the pepper and onion and cook gently, stirring, for 3–4 minutes until really soft but only lightly golden.

2 Beat the eggs with the water and a little salt and pepper. Pour into the pan and add the artichoke heart. Sprinkle the oregano and chilli flakes over.

3 Cook the omelette, lifting it at the edges as it sets, to allow the uncooked egg to run underneath.

4 When the under-side is golden brown and almost set, flash under a preheated grill (broiler) to brown the top.

5 Fold and serve garnished with a sprig of parsley.

Serves 1

Carbohydrates: 7 g

Dinner Starter Recipes

There is no more than a trace – that is, not even half a gram – of carbohydrates in a portion of any of these, so you can include them in a meal when you want a stylish, three-course dinner, or omit them when you don't need them.

Parma ham with marinated olives

This simple starter has an abundance of Mediterranean charm. You can make it with any cured pure meats if you prefer a change from traditional Parma ham.

1 Put all the ingredients except the ham in an airtight container with lid. Mix thoroughly, cover tightly and leave to marinate in the fridge for several hours or preferably overnight.

2 When ready to serve, arrange the ham in rippling folds on small plates. Discard the lemon zest and spoon the olives in a small pile to one side of the ham.

3 Garnish each plate with a wedge of lemon and a sprig of parsley or basil and serve.

175 g/6 oz mixed black and green stoned (pitted) olives

30 ml/2 tbsp olive oil

Thinly pared zest of ½ lemon

30 ml/2 tbsp dry white wine

1.5 ml/¼ tsp dried chilli flakes

A good grinding of black pepper

12 thin slices of Parma ham

4 wedges of lemon and 4 sprigs of fresh parsley or basil, for garnishing

Serves 4
Carbohydrates:
0 g per serving

Watercress roulade with cream cheese and chives

Pretty, light and elegant, this cool, green watercress roulade is rolled around a soft cheese and fresh chive filling, then served in slices with a nutty sesame dressing.

2 bunches of watercress

45 ml/3 tbsp grated Parmesan cheese

Salt and freshly ground black pepper

4 eggs, separated

225 g/8 oz/1 cup cream cheese

30 ml/2 tbsp snipped fresh chives

15 ml/1 tbsp full-fat soya milk

30 ml/2 tbsp sesame seeds

20 ml/4 tsp sesame oil

30 ml/2 tbsp olive oil

Serves 4
Carbohydrates: Trace per serving

1 Trim the feathery ends off the watercress stalks, then finely chop the leaves, preferably in a blender or food processor. Add 30 ml/2 tbsp of the Parmesan, a little salt and pepper and the egg yolks and beat well.

2 Whisk the egg whites until stiff, then fold in using a metal spoon.

3 Grease and line an 18 × 28 cm/ 7 × 11 in Swiss roll tin (jelly roll pan) with greased greaseproof (waxed) paper or non-stick baking parchment.

4 Spoon in the watercress mixture and spread out evenly. Bake in a preheated oven at 200°C/400°F/gas 6/fan oven 180°C for 12–15 minutes until risen and firm.

5 Lay another sheet of greaseproof paper or non-stick baking parchment on the work surface and dust with the remaining Parmesan. Turn the roulade out on to the sheet, loosen the cooking paper but leave in place, cover with a clean tea towel (dishcloth) and leave until cold.

6 Beat the cream cheese with the chives and soften slightly with a little soya milk. Season to taste.

7 Toast the sesame seeds in a frying pan (skillet) until golden, then tip out of the pan on to a saucer straight away to prevent burning.

8 Spread the cheese mixture over the cold roulade and roll up. Cut into eight slices and put two slices on each of four small plates.

9 Mix the sesame oil with the olive oil and trickle round the plates. Sprinkle round the plates with a few toasted sesame seeds and serve.

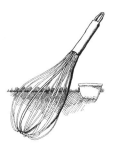

Smoked salmon with prawns and lemon

Thin slices of succulent smoked salmon, garnished with whole king prawns, fresh lemon and parsley make an elegant yet simple starter for any special occasion.

1 Arrange the slices of salmon on four plates with two prawns on the side of each.

2 Garnish with wedges of lemon and sprigs of parsley and serve with lots of freshly ground black pepper.

225 g/8 oz sliced smoked salmon

8 cooked unpeeled king prawns (jumbo shrimp)

Wedges of lemon and sprigs of fresh parsley, for garnishing

Freshly ground black pepper

Serves 4
Carbohydrates: 0 g

Individual baked eggs with pancetta

Another dish with a Mediterranean feel: the eggs are baked in individual pots over cubes of pancetta, first fried in olive oil, flavoured with fresh herbs and moistened with cream.

50 g/2 oz diced pancetta

15 ml/1 tbsp olive oil, plus extra for greasing

8 fresh sage or basil leaves, chopped

4 eggs

Freshly ground black pepper

60 ml/4 tbsp double (heavy) cream

4 small sprigs of fresh sage or basil, for garnishing

1 Grease four ramekin dishes (custard cups).

2 Fry (sauté) the pancetta in the olive oil for 2 minutes, stirring, until lightly golden but still soft.

3 Spoon the pancetta and the oil into the ramekin dishes. Sprinkle with the chopped sage or basil.

4 Break an egg into each pot and season with pepper. Spoon the cream over.

5 Stand the dishes in a baking tin (pan) containing enough boiling water to come halfway up the sides of the dishes. Bake the eggs in a preheated oven at 180°C/350°F/gas 4/fan oven 160°C for 10–15 minutes until cooked to your liking.

6 Place the ramekins on small plates and garnish each plate with a small sprig of fresh sage or basil.

Serves 4
Carbohydrates:
Trace per serving

Seafood and wild rocket salad

Prawns, squid, mussels and scallops piled on wild rocket and dressed with fragrant mayonnaise, olive oil and coriander. If you want to serve six, use wine goblets instead of plates.

1 Drain the seafood cocktail thoroughly on kitchen paper (paper towels).

2 Pile the rocket on four small plates.

3 Mix the dressing ingredients together and fold in the seafood cocktail.

4 Spoon on to the rocket and garnish each plate with a sprig of coriander and a wedge of lemon.

1 x 400 g/14 oz packet of frozen cooked seafood cocktail, just thawed

A good handful of wild rocket

For the dressing:

30 ml/2 tbsp mayonnaise

30 ml/2 tbsp olive oil

15 ml/1 tbsp lemon juice

10 ml/2 tsp chopped fresh coriander (cilantro)

Salt and freshly ground black pepper

Sprigs of coriander and wedges of lemon, for garnishing

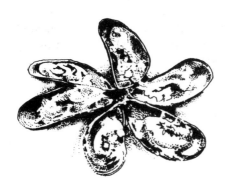

Serves 4
Carbohydrates: Trace

Sesame-fried Camembert on watercress

Wedges of Camembert, coated in sesame seeds and quickly fried until golden and gently melting in the middle, then served on a bed of watercress with a sesame oil dressing.

1 round of firm Camembert cheese, cut into 8 portions

1 egg, beaten

60 ml/4 tbsp sesame seeds

45 ml/3 tbsp olive oil

15 ml/1 tbsp sesame oil

15 ml/1 tbsp red wine vinegar

A good pinch of artificial sweetener

Salt and freshly ground black pepper

1 large bunch of watercress

Oil, for deep-frying

1 Dip each wedge of cheese in beaten egg, then sesame seeds, to coat completely. Repeat the coating if necessary. Chill until ready to cook.

2 Whisk the oils with the vinegar and season to taste with sweetener, salt and pepper.

3 Trim and discard the feathery stalks from the watercress. Put a pile of leaves in the centre of four small plates.

4 Heat the oil in a deep-fryer or deep pan to 190°C/375°F or until a few sesame seeds dropped into the oil rise to the surface, sizzle and brown within 30 seconds. Deep-fry the Camembert, in a frying basket if possible, for 1 minute until golden, turning over once if necessary.

5 Quickly place two wedges on each pile of watercress and trickle the dressing around the edge of the plates. Serve straight away.

Serves 4
Carbohydrates: Trace per serving

Carpaccio of beef with crushed black pepper

Wafer-thin slices of tender fillet steak, coated in crushed black peppercorns, drizzled with olive oil and lemon juice, topped with a few fresh Parmesan shavings and garnished with wild rocket.

1 Trim any sinews from the steak. Brush with 15 ml/1 tbsp of the olive oil, then roll in the peppercorns to coat thoroughly. Wrap in clingfilm (plastic wrap) and chill for at least 2 hours, then cut into thin slices.

2 Lay the slices side by side, two at a time, between sheets of clingfilm (plastic wrap) and beat with a meat mallet or the end of a rolling pin to flatten until wafer-thin.

3 Arrange the slices overlapping around the edge of four plates. Put a small pile of wild rocket in the centre of each.

4 Trickle the remaining olive oil and lemon juice over and scatter with the Parmesan shavings.

350 g/12 oz piece of thick fillet steak

75 ml/5 tbsp olive oil

10 ml/2 tsp crushed black peppercorns

50 g/2 oz wild rocket

15 ml/1 tbsp lemon juice

25 g/1 oz/¼ cup freshly shaved Parmesan cheese

Serves 4
Carbohydrates:
Trace per serving

King prawns in olive oil and garlic butter

Large prawns sautéed until just coral-pink in a glorious mixture of olive oil and unsalted butter, with garlic and chopped fresh parsley, served with wedges of lemon to offset the richness.

100 g/4 oz/'½ cup unsalted (sweet) butter

120 ml/4 fl oz/'½ cup olive oil

450 g/1 lb raw peeled king prawns (jumbo shrimp), tails left on

1 large garlic clove, crushed

30 ml/2 tbsp chopped fresh parsley

Wedges of lemon and sprigs of parsley, for garnishing

1 Melt a quarter of the butter and oil in a frying pan (skillet). Add the prawns and stir-fry for 2 minutes until just pink.

2 Add the remaining butter and oil, the garlic and parsley and allow to sizzle until melted.

3 Spoon the prawns and butter on to warm plates and garnish with wedges of lemon and sprigs of parsley. Serve straight away.

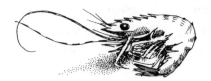

Serves 4

Carbohydrates: Trace per serving

Chilli-spiced scallops with bacon

If you use frozen scallops, allow them to defrost fully before use. Their sweet, mild flavour and succulent texture marry surprisingly well with chilli and bacon.

1 Cut the scallops into quarters.

2 Stretch each rasher of bacon with the back of a knife then cut in half lengthways.

3 Roll each piece of scallop in a piece of bacon and secure with a wooden cocktail stick (toothpick), if necessary.

4 Heat the oil in a frying pan (skillet) and fry (sauté) the scallop rolls for 2–3 minutes, turning until cooked through and golden all over.

5 Transfer the scallops to four warm plates. Remove the cocktail sticks, if necessary.

6 Add the chilli powder, a good grinding of pepper and the lemon juice to the oil in the pan and heat, stirring, until sizzling.

7 Pour the oil over the scallops and bacon, then garnish with wedges of lemon and sprigs of parsley to serve.

8 large, shelled fresh or frozen scallops

8 rashers (slices) of unsmoked streaky bacon, rinded

60 ml/4 tbsp olive oil

A pinch of chilli powder

Freshly ground black pepper

10 ml/2 tsp lemon juice

Wedges of lemon and little chopped parsley, for garnishing

Serves 4
Carbohydrates:
0 g per serving

Potted prawns with sweet spices

These are so easy to make and ideal for entertaining as you can prepare them in advance and chill them, ready to turn out, if you like, garnish and serve.

225 g/8 oz/1 cup unsalted (sweet) butter

450 g/1 lb cooked peeled prawns (shrimp)

1.5 ml/¼ tsp ground mace

A pinch of cayenne

Salt and freshly ground black pepper

Wedges of lemon and sprigs of parsley, for garnishing

1 Put half the butter in a saucepan and heat gently until melted.

2 Add the prawns and cook gently for 2 minutes until they are just heated through. Do not boil or the prawns will become tough.

3 Season to taste with the mace, cayenne, salt and pepper.

4 Pack into four small ramekins (custard cups).

5 Melt the remaining butter and pour over the top. Chill until firm.

6 Either serve in their pots or turn out on to small plates. Garnish with wedges of lemon and sprigs of parsley to serve.

Serves 4

Carbohydrates: 0 g per serving

Dinner Main Course Recipes

Each of the recipes in this section contains 10 g of carbohydrates and once again, you can mix and match your menus to suit your tastes – and appetite – on the day. They are imaginative enough to serve for guests, combined with one of the starters on pages 127–36, but you don't need a starter on ordinary evenings! Whatever you decide, do remember to make up your full carb allowance, using one of the desserts on pages 164–76 or extra vegetables from previous lists.

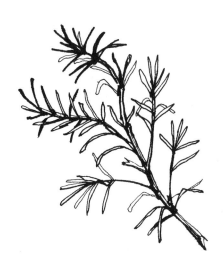

Poached salmon with baby vegetables

A selection of colourful baby vegetables, cooked until just tender, then served with a succulent salmon fillet poached in white wine and dressed in a watercress-flavoured Hollandaise sauce.

200 g/7 oz baby carrots

200 g/7 oz baby turnips

200 g/7 oz thin French (green) beans

200 g/7 oz baby corn cobs

200 g/7 oz mangetout (snow peas)

200 g/7 oz thin asparagus tips

4 pieces of salmon tail fillet, 175 g/6 oz each

150 ml/¼ pt/⅔ cup dry white wine

150 ml/¼ pt/⅔ cup water

1 bay leaf

1 onion, sliced

For the Hollandaise:

2 eggs

30 ml/2 tbsp lemon juice

100 g/4 oz/½ cup butter, melted

1 bunch of watercress

Salt and white pepper

Serves 4

Carbohydrates: 10 g per serving

1 Steam or boil all the vegetables. Cook the carrots and turnips for about 6 minutes, the beans and corn for about 4 minutes and the mangetout and asparagus for 2–3 minutes until they are all tender but still with some 'bite'. Drain, if necessary, and keep warm.

2 Meanwhile, put the fish in a shallow pan with the wine, water, bay leaf and onion. Bring to the boil, turn down the heat, cover and poach gently for 5–8 minutes, depending on thickness, until the fish can be separated easily into flakes with the point of a knife.

3 Make the Hollandaise. Whisk the eggs in a small, heavy-based saucepan. Whisk in the lemon juice. Gradually whisk in the melted butter. Cook over a gentle heat, whisking all the time until thickened. Do not allow to boil or the mixture will curdle. Trim and chop the watercress, stir in and season to taste.

4 Using a fish slice, carefully transfer the fish to four warmed plates. Arrange the vegetables in clusters around and spoon a little sauce over.

Chicken and vegetable stir-fry

For this recipe, tender chicken breast strips are stir-fried with a selection of vegetables, flavoured in oriental style with a dash of soy sauce, sherry and ginger.

1 Cut the chicken into thin strips. Cut the spring onions diagonally into short lengths. Cut the carrot and cucumber into matchsticks. Cut the peppers into thin strips.

2 Heat the oil in a large frying pan (skillet) or wok. Add the chicken and stir-fry for 3 minutes.

3 Add the spring onions, carrot, peppers and garlic and stir-fry for 2 minutes.

4 Add the cucumber, bamboo shoots and beansprouts and stir-fry for 1 minute.

5 Add the remaining ingredients and stir-fry for 1 minute.

6 Serve piled in warm bowls.

4 skinless chicken breasts

1 bunch of spring onions (scallions)

1 large carrot

10 cm/4 in piece of cucumber

30 ml/2 tbsp sunflower oil

1 green (bell) pepper

1 red pepper

1 garlic clove, crushed

1 x 225 g/8 oz/small can of bamboo shoots, drained

100 g/4 oz/2 cups beansprouts

30 ml/2 tbsp soy sauce

30 ml/2 tbsp dry sherry

2.5 ml/½ tsp ground ginger

2.5 ml/½ tsp artificial sweetener

Serves 4

Carbohydrates: 10 g per serving

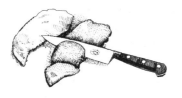

Chicken in red wine with mangetout and baby corn

Chicken cooked until meltingly tender with smoked lardons and garlic in a rich red wine sauce and served with mangetout, braised with onions and lettuce and sweet yellow baby corn.

15 ml/1 tbsp olive oil

50 g/2 oz smoked lardons (diced bacon)

1 garlic clove, crushed

4 chicken portions

600 ml/1 pt/2½ cups red wine

15 ml/1 tbsp tomato purée (paste)

15 ml/1 tbsp brandy

1 chicken stock cube

5 ml/1 tsp artificial sweetener

Salt and freshly ground black pepper

1 bouquet garni sachet

2 onions, each cut into 8 wedges

150 ml/¼ pt/⅔ cup water

15 g/½ oz/1 tbsp butter

1 Heat the oil in a large flameproof casserole dish (Dutch oven). Add the lardons and fry (sauté), stirring, for 1 minute. Add the garlic and cook for 1 further minute. Remove from the pan with a draining spoon.

2 Add the chicken to the pan and brown on all sides. Pour off any excess oil.

3 Return the lardons to the pan and add the wine and the tomato purée, blended with the brandy. Crumble in the stock cube and add the artificial sweetener, a little salt and pepper and the bouquet garni. Bring to the boil.

4 Cover the casserole, reduce the heat and simmer gently for 1 hour.

5 Meanwhile, put the onions in a saucepan with half the water and the butter. Cover and simmer for 3 minutes.

6 Add the remaining water, the mangetout, lettuce, mint and a sprinkling of salt and pepper.

7 Put the corn cobs in an even layer in a steamer or metal colander that will fit over the saucepan. Cover the top with a lid or foil and cook gently for 5 minutes, stirring once or twice until the corn cobs, mangetout and onions are tender. Remove the corn and keep warm. If necessary, boil the mangetout mixture rapidly, uncovered, for a minute or two to evaporate any water, stirring gently all the time.

8 When the chicken is cooked, carefully lift the portions out of the pan and keep warm. Boil the sauce rapidly until reduced by half. Discard the bouquet garni, taste and re-season if necessary.

9 Transfer the chicken to warm plates and spoon the sauce over. Sprinkle with the chopped parsley. Spoon the French-style mangetout and corn cobs to one side.

200 g/7 oz mangetout (snow peas)

1 round lettuce, shredded

5 ml/1 tsp dried mint

16 baby corn cobs

A little chopped fresh parsley, for garnishing

Serves 4

Carbohydrates: 10 g per serving

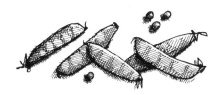

Mushroom-topped pork chops with red cabbage

Lean pork chops with a rich mushroom topping served on a bed of sweet and sour red cabbage and accompanied by golden-roasted baby leeks.

25 g/1 oz/2 tbsp butter

1 small red cabbage, shredded

1 red onion, halved and thinly sliced

Salt and freshly ground black pepper

30 ml/2 tbsp artificial sweetener

60 ml/4 tbsp red wine vinegar

30 ml/2 tbsp water

16 baby leeks, about 400 g/14 oz in weight, trimmed

450 ml/³⁄₄ pt/2 cups vegetable stock, made with 1 stock cube

30 ml/2 tbsp olive oil

4 large pork chops

4 large flat mushrooms, peeled and finely chopped

2.5 ml/½ tsp dried oregano

1 Melt the butter in a flameproof casserole dish (Dutch oven). Layer the cabbage and onion in the casserole, sprinkling each layer with a little salt and lots of pepper.

2 Mix the sweetener with the vinegar and water and pour over. Bring to the boil, cover tightly, then turn down the heat to very low and cook gently for 2 hours, stirring occasionally, until really tender.

3 Meanwhile, cook the leeks in the stock for 2 minutes only. Remove from the pan with a draining spoon and drain on kitchen paper (paper towels). Reserve the stock.

4 Heat half the oil in a frying pan (skillet). Fry (sauté) the leeks for 2 minutes, shaking the pan occasionally, until lightly golden. Remove from the pan and keep warm.

5 Season the chops on both sides with salt and pepper. Heat the remaining oil in the same pan and brown the chops quickly on both sides.

6 Turn down the heat to moderate and cook for 10 minutes until golden and cooked through, turning the chops once. Remove from the pan and keep warm.

7 Add the mushrooms to the oil in the pan and fry for 2 minutes, stirring. Add the reserved leek stock and the oregano, bring to the boil, stirring, then boil rapidly until well reduced and slightly syrupy, scraping up any sediment in the pan. Season to taste.

8 Transfer the red cabbage to warm plates, using a draining spoon to remove any excess moisture. Put the chops on top of the cabbage and spoon the sauce over. Arrange the leeks to one side and serve.

Serves 4
Carbohydrates:
10 g per serving

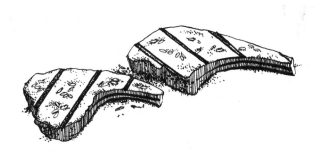

Nutty lamb chops with fresh mint jelly

Tender loin lamb chops in a nut and crumb coating, fried until pink and juicy, then served with stock-braised and mashed turnips and swede and shredded, lightly cooked spring greens.

150 ml/¼ pt/⅔ cup apple juice

5 ml/1 tsp powdered gelatine

45 ml/3 tbsp fresh chopped mint OR 10 ml/2 tsp dried mint

10 ml/2 tsp red wine vinegar

8 loin lamb chops

50 g/2 oz/½ cup chopped mixed nuts

4 slices of Low-carbohydrate Soya Bread (see page 113), crumbed

15 ml/1 tbsp chopped fresh parsley

2.5 ml/½ tsp dried oregano

A little salt and freshly ground black pepper

2 eggs, beaten

15 ml/1 tbsp olive oil

40 g/1½ oz/3 tbsp butter

1 small swede (rutabaga), cut into small chunks

4 turnips, cut into small chunks

1 Make the jelly well in advance to allow time to set. Put 30 ml/2 tbsp of the apple juice in a small bowl. Add the gelatine and leave to soften for 5 minutes. Stand the bowl in a pan of simmering water and stir until completely dissolved or heat briefly in the microwave. Stir in the remaining apple juice, the mint and vinegar. Turn into a small dish and chill.

2 Wipe the chops with kitchen paper (paper towels). Mix the nuts with the breadcrumbs, fresh and dried herbs and a little salt and pepper. Dip the chops in the beaten eggs, then the nut mixture, to coat completely. Chill until ready to cook.

3 Boil the swede and turnips in the stock for about 10 minutes or until really tender. Drain, reserving the stock. Put the vegetables back in the pan and mash with 30 ml/2 tbsp of the butter. Season well with pepper and stir in the crème fraîche. Keep warm.

4 Fry (sauté) the chops in the oil and half the remaining butter over a moderate heat for 4–5 minutes on each side until golden on the outside and pink in the centre. Remove from the pan and keep warm.

5 Cook the greens in 2.5 cm/1 in of boiling, lightly salted water for 3 minutes only. Drain the liquid into the lamb pan and keep the greens warm.

6 Pour the reserved swede and turnip stock into the lamb pan too. Boil rapidly, scraping up the sediment until well reduced and slightly thickened. Whisk in the last of the butter, a piece at a time. Season to taste.

7 Spoon the shredded greens on to warm plates. Top with the chops and spoon the sauce over. Serve with the vegetable mash and mint jelly.

600 ml/1 pt/2½ cups vegetable stock, made with 1 stock cube

15 ml/1 tbsp crème fraîche

450 g/1 lb spring (collard) greens, shredded

Serves 4
Carbohydrates: 10 g per serving

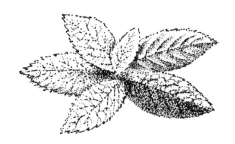

Warm duck breast salad with raspberries

Plump duck breasts served on a salad with toasted pine nuts and avocado, bathed in a warm dressing of fresh raspberries in olive oil and raspberry vinegar.

60 ml/4 tbsp pine nuts

100 g/4 oz mixed salad leaves

16 cherry tomatoes, halved

10 cm/4 in piece of cucumber, diced

4 spring onions (scallions), chopped

2 avocados

10 ml/2 tsp lemon juice

4 duck breasts, about 175 g/6 oz each

120 ml/4 fl oz/½ cup olive oil

45 ml/3 tbsp raspberry vinegar

30 ml/2 tbsp balsamic vinegar

Salt and freshly ground black pepper

2.5 ml/½ tsp artificial sweetener

100 g/4 oz fresh raspberries

1 Toast the pine nuts in a dry frying pan (skillet), then tip out of the pan immediately so they don't burn. Reserve.

2 Pile the salad leaves on large plates and scatter the pine nuts, tomatoes, cucumber and spring onions over.

3 Halve the avocados, remove the stones (pits), peel off the skin and dice the flesh. Toss in the lemon juice to prevent browning, then scatter over the salads.

4 Put the duck breasts, skin-sides down, on a board and remove the sinew that runs from the pointed end, using a sharp pointed knife. (This stops them curling up when cooked.) Season the duck-skin with salt and pepper.

5 Heat a large frying pan (skillet) add the duck, skin-sides down and fry (sauté) over a moderate heat for about 4 minutes until the fat runs and the skin is golden brown. Turn the duck over and cook for a further 4–6 minutes until cooked to your liking.

6 Remove from the pan, carefully take the skin off the duck, then wrap the breasts in foil and keep warm. Return the skin to the frying pan. Turn up the heat and cook until crisp, then remove and drain on kitchen paper (paper towels). Cut into shreds and reserve for garnishing.

7 Add the olive oil to the pan with the raspberry and balsamic vinegars. Bring to the boil, stirring and scraping up any sediment. Season the mixture with salt, pepper and the sweetener. Add the raspberries and stir to coat in the dressing.

8 Cut the duck breasts diagonally into slices and arrange on top of the salads. Spoon the dressing over and garnish with the crisp duck skin.

Serves 4

Carbohydrates:
10 g per serving

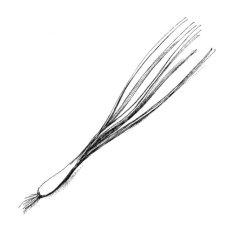

Steak with grainy mustard jus and beetroot chips

Thick, juicy sirloin steaks bathed in a white wine, brandy and crème fraîche sauce flavoured with grainy mustard, served with wafer-thin, deep-fried beetroot crisps and a cool green salad.

4 sirloin steaks, about 175 g/6 oz each

Salt and freshly ground black pepper

15 g/¹⁄₂ oz/1 tbsp butter

15 ml/1 tbsp olive oil

120 ml/4 fl oz/¹⁄₂ cup dry white wine

15 ml/1 tbsp grainy mustard

15 ml/1 tbsp brandy

120 ml/4 fl oz/¹⁄₂ cup crème fraîche

1.5 ml/¹⁄₄ tsp artificial sweetener

For the chips:

4 raw beetroot (red beets)

Oil, for deep-frying

1 Wipe the steaks and season with salt and pepper. Fry in the butter and oil for 2 minutes on each side to brown, then turn down the heat and cook for a further 4–10 minutes until cooked to your liking, turning once. Remove from the pan and keep warm.

2 Add the wine to the pan and boil until reduced by half. Stir in the mustard, brandy, crème fraîche and sweetener and season to taste. Remove from the heat.

3 Meanwhile, make the beetroot chips. Peel the beetroot and cut into very thin slices with a mandolin slicer or a very sharp knife. Wipe on kitchen paper (paper towels).

4 Deep-fry the slices in hot oil for about 2¹⁄₂ minutes until crisp and turning orange-pink. Don't cook any longer or they will burn. Drain on kitchen paper. Keep warm.

5 Arrange the salad ingredients in small bowls. Whisk the oil and vinegar together and drizzle over. Season with lots of pepper.

6 Transfer the steaks to warm plates and spoon the sauce over. Garnish with the chopped parsley. Pile the chips to one side and serve with the salad.

For the salad:

¼ iceberg lettuce, torn into small pieces

1 bunch of watercress, trimmed and separated into small sprigs

4 spring onions (scallions), cut into short lengths

1 box of salad cress

45 ml/3 tbsp olive oil

15 ml/1 tbsp balsamic vinegar

15 ml/1 tbsp chopped fresh parsley, for garnishing

Serves 4

Carbohydrates: 10 g per serving

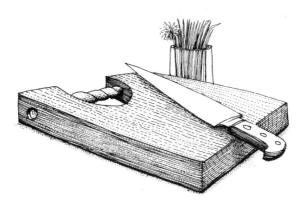

Thai prawn and cucumber curry with wild rice

Subtle flavours of lemon grass and coconut with garlic, spring onions and a selection of sweet and hot spices are blended together in this creamy curry, packed with king prawns.

225 g/8 oz/1 cup wild rice

1 cucumber, quartered lengthways and cut into bite-sized chunks

15 g/½ oz/1 tbsp butter

2 garlic cloves, crushed

5 ml/1 tsp grated fresh root ginger

1 stalk of lemon grass, finely chopped

1 bunch of spring onions (scallions), finely chopped

5 ml/1 tsp ground turmeric

10 ml/2 tsp garam masala

1.5 ml/¼ tsp ground cloves

2.5 ml/½ tsp ground cinnamon

2 green chillies, seeded and finely chopped

5 ml/1 tsp artificial sweetener

1 Cook the wild rice in boiling, lightly salted water for 20–30 minutes until just tender but still with some 'bite'. Drain and keep warm.

2 Meanwhile, put the cucumber in a pan with just enough water to cover. Add a pinch of salt. Bring to the boil, reduce the heat and simmer for 5 minutes. Drain.

3 Melt the butter in a saucepan. Add the garlic, ginger, lemon grass, spring onions, all the spices and the chillies. Cook, stirring, for 1 minute.

4 Add the sweetener, coconut and stock. Bring to the boil and simmer, stirring all the time, until the coconut melts.

5 Add the prawns and cucumber and simmer for 5 minutes, stirring. Season to taste.

6 Pile the rice into warm bowls and spoon the curry over. Garnish each with a few chive stalks and serve.

Note: You must use pure wild rice for this recipe, not wild rice mix, a combination of wild rice and long-grain rice that has a high carbohydrate content.

100 g/4 oz/½ block of creamed coconut, cut into chunks

450 ml/¾ pt/2 cups fish stock, made with 1 stock cube

400 g/14 oz raw peeled king prawns (jumbo shrimp), split in half lengthways

Salt and freshly ground black pepper

A few fresh chive stalks, for garnishing

Serves 4
Carbohydrates: 10 g per serving

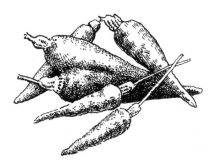

Turkey, ham and cheese rolls with tomato coulis

Thinly beaten turkey steaks, rolled up with sweet-cured cooked ham and melting cheese, sautéed until golden, then sliced and served on a bed of shredded omelette with a rich tomato sauce.

4 turkey breast steaks, about 175 g/6 oz each

4 slices of ham

4 slices of Leerdammer or Emmental (Swiss) cheese

For the coulis:

1 red onion, finely chopped

30 ml/2 tbsp olive oil

1 garlic clove, crushed

1 x 400 g/14 oz/large can of chopped tomatoes

15 ml/1 tbsp tomato purée (paste)

Salt and freshly ground black pepper

1.5 ml/¼ tsp artificial sweetener

15 ml/1 tbsp chopped fresh basil

For the omelette tagliatelle:

2 eggs

30 ml/2 tbsp water

2.5 ml/½ tsp Italian seasoning

1 Put the steaks one at a time in a plastic bag and beat with a rolling pin or meat mallet to flatten.

2 Lay a slice of ham and a slice of cheese on each steak and roll up. Secure each with a wooden cocktail stick (toothpick).

3 Make the coulis. Fry (sauté) the onion in the olive oil for 2 minutes, stirring. Add the garlic, tomatoes and tomato purée. Bring to the boil, stirring, then reduce the heat and simmer for about 5 minutes, stirring occasionally. Season to taste and stir in the sweetener and basil. Remove from the heat.

4 Make the omelette tagliatelle. Beat the eggs and water together, then beat in a little salt and pepper and the Italian seasoning.

5 Heat half the butter and olive oil in an omelette pan. Pour in half the egg mixture and cook, lifting the edge to allow the uncooked egg to run underneath. Do not stir, as you would when cooking an omelette – the mixture should remain flat.

6 When golden underneath and almost set, flip the omelette over and cook the other side, then slide out on to a plate and roll up. Repeat with the remaining, butter, oil and egg mixture. Cover the plate with foil and keep warm.

7 Arrange all the salad stuffs in four small salad bowls. Whisk the oil, vinegar, sweetener and a good pinch each of salt and pepper together and drizzle over the salads.

8 Finally, cook the turkey rolls. Heat a little oil in a frying pan (skillet). Add the turkey rolls and fry (sauté), turning occasionally for 8 minutes until cooked through and golden. Reheat the coulis.

9 Cut the omelette rolls into thin slices, then arrange the shreds in a pile on each of four warm plates. Remove the cocktail sticks from the turkey, cut each roll into six slices and arrange beside the omelette tagliatelle. Spoon a little coulis over, garnish with sprigs of basil and serve straight away.

25 g/1 oz/2 tbsp butter

30 ml/2 tbsp olive oil

For the salad:

1 round lettuce, torn into pieces

4 canned artichoke hearts, quartered

10 cm/4 in piece of cucumber, cut into small dice

4 spring onions (scallions), trimmed and chopped

45 ml/3 tbsp olive oil

15 ml/1 tbsp red wine vinegar

2.5 ml/½ tsp Dijon mustard

2.5 ml/½ tsp artificial sweetener

A little oil, for cooking

Fresh sprigs of basil, for garnishing

Serves 4

Carbohydrate: 10 g per serving

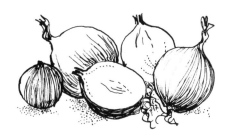

Poussins with pesto and Italian roasted vegetables

Pesto sauce has less than 1 g of carbohydrate per serving, so you can enjoy this recipe as a flavouring for all sorts of dishes as well as this delicious one with poussins and roasted vegetables.

For the pesto:

20 fresh basil leaves

1 large sprig of fresh parsley

50 g/2 oz/½ cup pine nuts

1 garlic clove, crushed

75 ml/5 tbsp olive oil

30 ml/2 tbsp freshly grated Parmesan cheese

Salt and freshly ground black pepper

For the poussins:

4 poussins (Cornish hens)

15 ml/1 tbsp olive oil

For the vegetables:

1 red (bell) pepper, cut into wide strips

1 green pepper, cut into wide strips

2 courgettes (zucchini), cut diagonally into slices

1 aubergine (eggplant), sliced

5 ml/1 tsp dried rosemary, crushed

1 Make the pesto. Put the herbs, pine nuts and garlic in a blender or food processor. Run the machine briefly to chop. With the machine running, gradually add the oil in a trickle to form a thick paste. Stop and scrape down the sides as necessary. Add the cheese, and season to taste and run the machine to form a well-flavoured paste.

2 Wipe the poussins inside and out with kitchen paper. Loosen the skin round the breast cavity end and smear the pesto between the skin and the flesh. Place in a roasting tin (pan). Rub all over with the olive oil and season the breasts with a fine sprinkling of salt, if liked.

3 Put all the prepared vegetables in a roasting tin. Sprinkle with the rosemary and the olive oil. Season with lots of pepper and toss with your hands so that all the vegetables are coated in the oil, then spread out in an even layer.

4 Put the poussins in the centre of a preheated oven at 180°C/350°F/ gas 4/fan oven 160°C for 15 minutes.

5 Put the vegetables at the top of the oven and roast for a further 20–30 minutes or until the vegetables and poussins are tender.

6 Transfer the poussins and the vegetables to warm plates. Spoon the poussins' roasting juices over. Garnish the plates with sprigs of parsley before serving.

90 ml/6 tbsp olive oil

Sprigs of fresh parsley, for garnishing

Serves 4

Carbohydrates: 10 g per serving

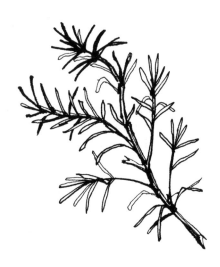

155

Lunchtime Desserts and Savouries

All these simply delicious desserts have 3 g of carbohydrates. If you prefer something savoury, you can always just have cheese with a breadstick, or some celery and a tomato, for your carb allowance. Alternatively, if you don't feel like having an extra course, have more salad or vegetables with your main course (see the list on page 102).

Creamy fresh gooseberry ripple

A simple fool that is delicious at any time. You can make a larger quantity and store it in the fridge to eat over the next few days. You can also substitute rhubarb if you can't get gooseberries.

100 g/4 oz gooseberries, topped and tailed

15 ml/1 tbsp water

A few drops of green food colouring (optional)

Artificial sweetener

45 ml/3 tbsp double (heavy) cream

1 Put the gooseberries in a pan with the water. Cover and cook over a fairly gentle heat until pulpy.

2 Stir in a few drops of food colouring, if liked, and sweeten to taste. Beat well with a wooden spoon until fairly smooth. Leave until cold.

3 Whip the cream and fold into the fruit purée, just enough to give a marbled effect. Spoon into a glass and serve.

Serves 1
Carbohydrates: 3 g

Raspberry crush cream

You could use blackberries instead of raspberries for another simple yet gorgeous dessert. Use a teaspoon of finely grated lemon zest for extra tang.

1 Reserve one raspberry for decoration. Put the remainder in a bowl and add the lemon juice. Crush with a fork so they are roughly mashed but not pulpy. Sweeten to taste with artificial sweetener.

2 Add the crème fraîche and fold through the raspberries. Spoon into a wine glass and decorate the top with the reserved raspberry. Chill until ready to serve.

1 heaped tbsp fresh or thawed frozen raspberries

A squeeze of lemon juice

Artificial sweetener

75 ml/5 tbsp crème fraîche

Serves 1
Carbohydrates: 3 g

Devils and angels on horseback

Sweet olive-stuffed prune halves (devils) and tender mushrooms (angels), wrapped in bacon and cooked until golden. The angels have no carbs so you can eat as many as you like but two devils are your limit!

1 Put an olive in each half prune. Place each on a piece of bacon and roll up. Secure with wooden cocktail sticks (toothpicks). Repeat with the mushrooms.

2 Grill (broil) or fry (sauté) the rolls, turning occasionally, until the bacon is browned all over.

3 Serve hot or cold.

2 stuffed olives

1 ready-to-eat prune, halved

2 button mushrooms, halved

3 rashers (slices) of streaky bacon, rinded and halved

Serves 1
Carbohydrates: 3 g

Chocolate cheese with walnuts

This smooth, velvety chocolate dessert has the added crunchy texture and complementary flavour of walnuts to help offset the richness.

10 ml/2 tsp cocoa (unsweetened chocolate) powder

10 ml/2 tsp boiling water

50 g/2 oz/¼ cup cream cheese

10 ml/2 tsp artificial sweetener

45 ml/3 tbsp double (heavy) cream, whipped

30 ml/2 tbsp walnuts, chopped

1 Blend the cocoa with the boiling water to form a smooth paste.

2 Stir in the cheese and sweetener, then fold in the whipped cream and half the walnuts.

3 Spoon the mixture into a small glass dish and top with the remaining walnuts. Chill until ready to serve.

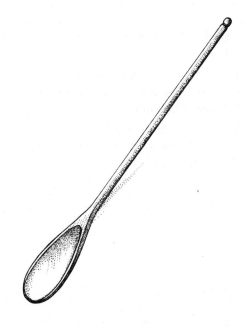

Serves 1
Carbohydrates: 3 g

Citrus jelly with fresh clementines

Another simple but effective way of making a sugar-free jelly into a delectable dessert. The lemon juice just sharpens and accentuates the refreshing flavour.

1 Thinly pare the zest off one of the clementines and cut it into thin strips. Boil in water for 2 minutes, then drain, rinse with cold water, drain again and reserve. Peel both the clementines, separate into segments, then cut into small pieces.

2 Put the fruit in four large wine goblets.

3 Make up the jelly according to the packet directions, reducing the quantity of water by 15 ml/1 tbsp and adding the lemon juice to the mixture. Leave to cool.

4 When the jelly is cold but not set, pour over the fruit in the glasses and stir well. Chill until set.

5 Top with a teaspoonful of crème fraîche and decorate with the reserved clementine zest.

2 clementines

1 packet of orange sugar-free jelly (jello) crystals

15 ml/1 tbsp lemon juice

20 ml/4 tsp crème fraîche

Serves 4
Carbohydrates:
3 g per serving

Creamy mousse with fresh strawberries

The crushed strawberries, eggs and cream in this scrumptious dessert lift it into the gourmet class! It's not worth bothering to make for one person, but it will keep in the fridge for a few days.

1 packet of sugar-free strawberry jelly (jello) crystals

150 ml/¼ pt/⅔ cup boiling water

175 g/6 oz strawberries, hulled

2 eggs, separated

120 ml/4 fl oz /½ cup double (heavy) cream

1 Dissolve the jelly crystals in the boiling water. Make up to 300 ml/ ½ pt/1¼ cups with cold water.

2 Reserve four slices of strawberry for decoration. Purée the remainder in a blender or food processor. Whisk in the egg yolks and the jelly.

3 Chill the mixture until it has the consistency of egg white, then whisk the egg whites until stiff and the cream until peaking.

4 Fold the cream, then the egg whites into the strawberry mixture and turn into a glass dish. Chill until set and decorate with the strawberry slices before serving.

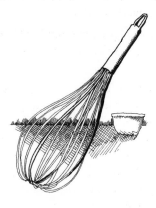

Serves 4

Carbohydrates: 3 g per serving

Coffee honeycomb mould with pecans

The mixture separates to form a clear jelly with a fluffy mousse on top. Smothered in cream and topped with pecans, it makes a fabulous end to your meal.

1 Put the egg yolks and sweetener in a bowl and whisk until thick and pale.

2 Warm the milk until almost boiling, then stir into the egg yolks. Pour back into the saucepan and cook over a gentle heat, stirring all the time, until the mixture thickens slightly. Do not allow to boil.

3 Sprinkle the gelatine over 45 ml/ 3 tbsp of the water in a small bowl and leave to soften for 5 minutes. Stand the bowl in a pan of hot water and stir until completely dissolved. Alternatively, heat briefly in the microwave but do not allow to boil.

4 Blend the coffee with the remaining water and stir into the custard with the dissolved gelatine.

5 Whisk the egg whites until stiff and fold into the mixture with a metal spoon.

6 Spoon into four large wine glasses or a lightly oiled jelly mould and chill until set. Put a spoonful of whipped cream on top of each individual glass and decorate with the pecan halves or turn out the mould and decorate with the nuts round the edge and serve with the whipped cream.

2 eggs, separated

60 ml/4 tbsp artificial sweetener

300 ml/½ pt/1¼ cups fortified unsweetened soya milk

10 ml/2 tsp powdered gelatine

90 ml/6 tbsp water

15 ml/1 tbsp instant coffee granules

60 ml/4 tbsp double (heavy) cream, whipped

30 ml/2 tbsp pecan nuts

Serves 4

Carbohydrates: 3 g per serving

Creamy yoghurt with hazelnuts

The full flavour of toasted hazelnuts permeates the sweetened blend of yoghurt and crème fraîche to make a fabulous, tasty dessert with a lovely contrast of textures.

60 ml/4 tbsp plain Greek-style strained cows' milk yoghurt

60 ml/4 tbsp crème fraîche

15 ml/1 tbsp water

15 ml/1 tbsp toasted chopped hazelnuts (filberts)

5 ml/1 tsp artificial sweetener

1 whole hazelnut, for decoration

1 Mix the yoghurt with the crème fraîche and water. Stir in the chopped hazelnuts and add sweetener to taste.

2 Chill for at least 1 hour (preferably longer) to allow the flavours to develop.

3 Decorate with a whole hazelnut before eating.

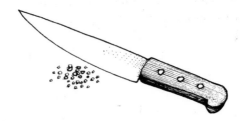

Serves 1
Carbohydrates: 3 g

Light and lacy soya crêpes with lemon

These low-carb crêpes can be served hot or cold, and stuffed with sweet or savoury fillings, as you would with ordinary pancakes. They can also be shredded instead of pasta and freeze well.

1 Mix the flour and salt in a bowl.

2 Whisk in the milk, water and eggs to form a smooth batter.

3 Heat a little oil in an omelette pan and pour off the excess. Add enough batter to just coat the base when it is swirled around. Cook until golden underneath, then flip over and cook the other side. Slide out of the pan and keep warm on a plate over a pan of hot water while you cook the remainder in the same way.

4 Smear each serving with a small knob of butter and add a sprinkling of sweetener and a squeeze of lemon juice. Roll up and serve.

For the pancakes:

50 g/2 oz/½ cup full-fat soya flour

A pinch of salt

75 ml/5 tbsp fortified unsweetened soya milk

75 ml/5 tbsp water

3 large eggs

Sunflower oil, for cooking

To finish:

Butter, artificial sweetener and lemon juice

Serves 4 (12 small pancakes)

Carbohydrates: 3 g per serving

After-dinner Desserts and Savouries

These mouth-watering, seductive desserts all contain 5 g of carbohydrates. If you prefer, you can have a portion of fruit or nuts to the same carbohydrate value (see pages 101–2). Alternatively, if you don't want a sweet, have cheese, a bread stick and a tomato, or have extra salad or vegetables to the same value with your main course.

Fresh lychees with ripe French Brie

This hardly seems to warrant a recipe, but these translucent sweet fruit deserve to be better known. They are the perfect accompaniment to just-ripe Brie to round off a meal.

5 fresh lychees
A large wedge of Brie

1 Peel the lychees by squeezing them gently. They should simply pop out of their skins if they are ripe.
2 Cut each fruit in half, if liked, and remove the stone (pit). Arrange on a plate with the cheese and serve.

Serves 1
Carbohydrates: 5 g

Strawberry and Greek yoghurt sesame brûlée

A brûlée is normally made with burnt sugar, but here I use toasted sesame seeds to give a golden, crisp top over plump juicy strawberries under sweetened cream and strained yoghurt.

1 Put the strawberries in the base of four ramekin dishes (custard cups).

2 Whip the yoghurt with the cream, vanilla and sweetener until thick. Spoon the mixture over the strawberries and chill until ready to serve.

3 Preheat the grill (broiler). Sprinkle the tops liberally with the sesame seeds and grill (broil) until golden. Serve straight away.

225 g/8 oz strawberries, hulled and sliced

100 ml/3½ fl oz/scant ½ cup plain Greek-style strained cows' milk yoghurt

150 ml/¼ pt/⅔ cup double (heavy) cream

2.5 ml/½ tsp vanilla essence (extract)

30 ml/2 tbsp artificial sweetener

60 ml/4 tbsp sesame seeds

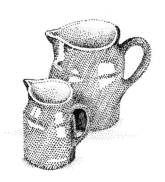

Serves 4
Carbohydrates:
5 g per serving

Hazelnut cream with raspberry coulis

A delicious nutty set cream with a smooth raspberry sauce, this is ideal for entertaining. If eating alone, make half the quantity and enjoy it two days running.

25 g/1 oz/¼ cup hazelnuts (filberts)

2 eggs

450 ml/¾ pt/2 cups double (heavy) cream

30 ml/2 tbsp artificial sweetener

A few drops of vanilla essence (extract)

A little oil, for greasing

For the coulis:

175 g/6 oz fresh raspberries

A pinch of artificial sweetener

A squeeze of lemon juice

Small sprigs of fresh mint, for decoration

1 Finely grind the hazelnuts in a blender or food processor.

2 Whisk the eggs, then whisk in the cream and sweeten with the artificial sweetener and vanilla. Stir in the nuts.

3 Lightly oil four ramekin dishes (custard cups). Pour in the cream mixture. Place in frying pan (skillet) with enough boiling water to come halfway up the sides of the dishes. Cover the pan with a lid or foil and simmer over a very low heat for about 30 minutes until set. Do not heat quickly or the mixture will curdle.

4 Remove the dishes from the pan, leave to cool, then chill.

5 Meanwhile, make the coulis. Purée the raspberries in a blender or food processor and sweeten to taste. Sharpen with a squeeze of lemon juice. Pass the mixture through a fine sieve (strainer) into a bowl. Chill.

6 When ready to serve, loosen the edges and turn the creams out on to small plates. Trickle the raspberry coulis around and decorate each with a small sprig of mint.

Serves 4

Carbohydrates: 5 g per serving

Mandarin orange cheese sherbet

A frozen dessert of cottage cheese blended with freshly squeezed mandarin orange juice and a hint of spices to make a delicious low-carbohydrate dessert fit for any occasion.

1 Grate the zest of one of the mandarins, thinly pare the zest from the other and squeeze the juice from both. Cut the pared zest into thin strips and boil in water for 2 minutes. Drain, rinse and drain again.

2 Blend the grated zest, juice, cheese, sweetener and spice until smooth. Alternatively pass the cheese through a fine sieve (strainer) and beat in the remaining ingredients.

3 Turn the mixture into a shallow freezer-proof container, cover with foil, and freeze for 2 hours. Whisk with a fork to break up the ice crystals.

4 Whisk the egg white until stiff and fold into the mixture with a metal spoon. Re-cover and return to the freezer. Freeze for a further 1½ hours. Whisk with a fork again to break up the ice crystals then freeze until firm.

5 When ready to serve, scoop the mixture into wine goblets and sprinkle with the thinly pared mandarin zest.

2 mandarin oranges

225 g/8 oz/1 cup cottage cheese

30 ml/2 tbsp artificial sweetener

A pinch of ground mixed (apple-pie) spice

1 egg white

Serves 4
Carbohydrates:
5 g per serving

167

Apricot Zabaglione with saffron buns

This traditional Italian dessert is a fluffy, warm concoction of eggs and sherry. I have added apricots and served it with a saffron bun. Freeze extra buns or store in an airtight container.

For the buns:

1.5 ml/¼ tsp saffron strands

10 ml/2 tsp boiling water

A little oil, for greasing

4 eggs, separated

90 ml/6 tbsp artificial sweetener, plus extra for dusting

75 g/3 oz/¾ cup full-fat soya flour

20 ml/4 tsp baking powder

50 g/2 oz/¼ cup butter, melted

60 ml/4 tbsp crème fraîche

15 ml/1 tbsp poppy seeds

4 ready-to-eat dried apricots

For the zabaglione:

2 eggs

30 ml/2 tbsp artificial sweetener

45 ml/3 tbsp dry sherry

1 Infuse the saffron in the water for 30 minutes.

2 Grease the 12 sections of a tartlet tin (patty pan) or line them with paper cases (cupcake papers).

3 Whisk the egg yolks with the sweetener until thick. Sift the flour and baking powder over the surface and fold in with the butter, infused saffron and crème fraîche.

4 Whisk the egg whites until stiff and fold in with a metal spoon.

5 Spoon the mixture into the prepared tins or paper cases, sprinkle with the poppy seeds and bake in a preheated oven at 180°C/350°F/gas 4/fan oven 160°C for about 8 minutes until risen and golden. Leave to cool slightly, then remove from the tin and cool on a wire rack.

6 Put the apricots in a pan and add just enough water to cover. Bring to the boil, turn down the heat and simmer gently for 10 minutes until really soft. If necessary, turn up the heat and boil rapidly, uncovered, to evaporate most of the liquid. Leave the fruit to cool, then snip into small pieces with scissors.

7 When nearly ready to serve, make the zabaglione. Break the eggs into a bowl. Add the sweetener and sherry.

8 Stand the bowl over a pan of gently simmering water and whisk, preferably with an electric beater, until thick and fluffy. Spoon the fruit into four wine glasses and top with the warm zabaglione. Serve each with a saffron bun.

Serves 4

Carbohydrates: 5 g per serving (including 2 g for 1 saffron bun)

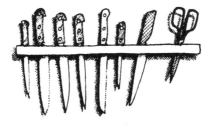

Fromage blanc with hot plum sauce

A cool, white mound of fresh cheese, bathed in a rich, sharp, fresh plum sauce. Use Quark instead of fromage blanc, if you prefer, in this simple dessert.

10 small plums, halved and stoned (pitted)

30 ml/2 tbsp water

Artificial sweetener, to taste

225 g/8 oz/1 cup fromage blanc

1 Put the plums in a pan with the water. Bring to the boil, turn down the heat, cover and cook gently until tender and pulpy.

2 Purée the plums in a blender or food processor, return to the pan and sweeten to taste with artificial sweetener. Reheat but do not boil.

3 Spoon the fromage blanc in a pile on each of four small plates. Trickle the hot plum sauce around and serve straight away.

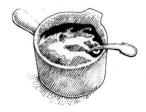

Serves 4

Carbohydrates: 5 g per serving

Potted Stilton with red wine and fennel

A wonderful end to any gourmet meal: ripe Stilton cheese, blended with butter and spices, moistened with red wine and packed in pots. Serve with cool fennel and crisp breadsticks.

1 Discard any rind on the cheese. Mash with half the butter, the spices, mustard and wine until well blended. Pack the mixture into four small pots.

2 Melt the remaining butter. Pour a little over the top of each pot, leaving the sediment behind. Press a sage leaf and 3 juniper berries into the butter, so they are coated. Leave to cool, then chill.

3 Trim the fennel, cut into quarters lengthways and separate into pieces. Put a pot of Stilton on each of four plates and serve with the fennel pieces and one breadstick per serving.

175 g/6 oz ripe Stilton

250 g/9 oz/good 1 cup butter, softened

1.5 ml/¼ tsp ground mace

1.5 ml/¼ tsp paprika

1.5 ml/¼ tsp made English mustard

45 ml/3 tbsp red wine

12 juniper berries

4 sage leaves

2 heads of fennel

4 crisp Italian breadsticks

Serves 4
Carbohydrates:
5 g per serving

171

Apricot and persimmon melba

Apricots stuffed with Mascarpone, surrounded by a sweet but tangy persimmon sauce and decorated with toasted almonds. You can use 200 g/7 oz raspberries instead of the persimmon.

1 ripe persimmon (Sharon fruit)

60 ml/4 tbsp water

10 ml/2 tsp lemon juice

A few drops of red food colouring (optional)

50 g/2 oz/4 tbsp Mascarpone cheese

Artificial sweetener, to taste

4 fresh apricots, halved and stoned (pitted)

30 ml/2 tbsp toasted flaked (slivered) almonds

1 Remove the stalk from the persimmon and roughly chop the fruit. Place in a saucepan with half the water. Bring to the boil, cover and cook gently for 7–10 minutes or until pulpy.

2 Purée in a blender or food processor or rub through a sieve (strainer), then add the remaining water and the lemon juice.

3 Mash the cheese with a little sweetener to taste and spoon into the apricots.

4 Spoon the persimmon sauce into four dishes. Place two apricot halves on top.

5 Chill until ready to serve sprinkled with the almonds.

Serves 4

Carbohydrates: 5 g per serving

Blackcurrant dream with orange zest

This dessert is made with blackcurrants, cooked gently with orange zest, then layered with a fluffy blend of strained yoghurt and crème fraîche.

1 Reserve four blackcurrants for decoration. Put the remainder in a saucepan with the water and orange zest and stew until the juice runs. Simmer gently to evaporate most of the juice, stirring occasionally. The fruit should now be soft but still have some shape. Stir in 30 ml/2 tbsp of the sweetener. Leave to cool.

2 Whisk the egg whites until stiff.

3 Mix the yoghurt with the crème fraîche and remaining sweetener, then fold in the whisked egg whites.

4 Layer the stewed fruit and fluffy yoghurt cream in four glasses, finishing with a layer of yoghurt mixture. Decorate the tops with the reserved fruits and tiny sprigs of mint. Chill until ready to serve.

200 g/7 oz fresh or frozen blackcurrants

120 ml/4 fl oz/½ cup water

5 ml/1 tsp finely grated orange zest

45 ml/3 tbsp artificial sweetener

2 egg whites

120 ml/4 fl oz/½ cup plain Greek-style strained cows' milk yoghurt

120 ml/4 fl oz/½ cup crème fraîche

4 tiny sprigs of fresh mint

Serves 4
Carbohydrates:
5 g per serving

Avocado whip with a dash of lime

A delicious sweet way of serving avocado, this makes a creamy mousse with a delicate flavour. You can poach the egg yolks in a little water and use them, sieved, to garnish savoury dishes.

1 lime

2 ripe avocados

30 ml/2 tbsp artificial sweetener

2 egg whites

250 ml/8 fl oz/1 cup double (heavy) cream

1 Thinly pare the zest from the lime and cut it into thin strips. Boil in water for 2 minutes. Drain, rinse with cold water and drain again.

2 Squeeze the lime juice into a bowl.

3 Halve the avocados, remove the stones (pits) and scoop the flesh into the lime juice. Mash thoroughly with a fork until smooth. Sweeten to taste with artificial sweetener.

4 Whisk the egg whites until stiff and the cream until peaking. Fold about three-quarters of the cream into the avocado mixture, then fold in the egg whites with a metal spoon. Spoon into glasses and top with a spoonful of the remaining cream.

5 Sprinkle with the blanched lime rind and chill for an hour to firm before serving.

Serves 4

Carbohydrates: 5 g per serving

Low-carbohydrate Italian tiramisu

Low-carb bread instead of sponge cake makes this an ideal dessert. The name means 'pick-me-up' and it will do that with its coffee-and-brandy base beneath cool Mascarpone and cream.

1 Put the bread slices in the base of four individual dishes. Mix the water with the coffee until dissolved and sweeten with 20 ml/4 tsp of the artificial sweetener. Stir in half the brandy. Spoon over the bread to cover completely and mash with a fork to soak in thoroughly.

2 Beat the Mascarpone with the remaining brandy and the remaining sweetener. Spread over the coffee mixture.

3 Cover with whipped cream and dust with a sprinkling of cinnamon. Chill until ready to serve.

4 slices of Low-carbohydrate Soya Bread (see page 113)

120 ml/4 fl oz/½ cup hot water

15 ml/1 tbsp instant coffee granules

30 ml/ 2 tbsp artificial sweetener

45 ml/3 tbsp brandy

225 g/8 oz/1 cup Mascarpone cheese

150 ml/¼ pt/⅔ cup double (heavy) cream, whipped

A little ground cinnamon, for dusting

Serves 4
Carbohydrates:
5 g per serving

Whisky lemon syllabub with coconut dusting

Creamy and sharp yet sweet, with a little shot of whisky for added kick and a dusting of toasted coconut for texture, this dessert is a wonderful twist on an old favourite.

Finely grated rind and juice of 1 lemon

30 ml/2 tbsp artificial sweetener

30 ml/2 tbsp whisky

250 ml/8 fl oz/1 cup single (light) cream

250 ml/8 fl oz/1 cup crème fraîche

15 ml/1 tbsp toasted desiccated (shredded) coconut, for decoration

1 Mix the lemon rind and juice with the sweetener and whisky until dissolved.

2 Add the creams and whisk until softly peaking. Spoon into four wine goblets and chill for at least 2 hours.

3 Serve sprinkled with the coconut.

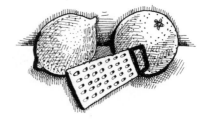

Serves 4

Carbohydrates: 5 g per serving

Phase 3: Time for Treats

When you've nearly lost all the weight you need to – it may be after a few weeks, or it may be much longer – you can move on to Phase 3 of the plan. You are probably already having at least 45–50 g of carbohydrate per day, maybe more, and are still losing weight slowly, so now is the time to introduce a few carbohydrate 'treats' – in moderation. You may be feeling really fit and healthy, but this makes this phase all the more tricky because, as you are able to indulge in a few extras, it is easy to go over the top. But with that word 'moderation' in mind, you will reach your goal. It may take a few weeks, it may take several months but then, ideally, you will be completely equipped to maintain your weight and enjoy your food for the rest of your life.

Hitting a plateau

You've been on the diet for a few weeks, and everything has been going well, with your weight slowly dropping. Then suddenly, you hit an impasse as, for no apparent reason, the weight loss stops. Don't worry, this is something that happens to many people sooner or later before they reach their goal. Providing you are not actually gaining weight, your carbohydrate levels are about right. However, if your weight is going up again, you need to cut back on the carbohydrates, starting with the treats in this section (see the advice on the next pages). Don't cut out the essential low-carbohydrate fruit and veggies.

Don't worry until the plateau has continued for more than three or four weeks. Your body may just be readjusting to the new phase of the diet and, providing you don't give up the regime, you will begin to lose weight again. Also, check your measurements. If you've lost in size all you wanted, you may already have reached your goal, even if it is a couple of kilos/pounds heavier than you'd originally planned.

If, however, you still have a little bit to lose and it won't budge, try one of the following ways to re-start your weight loss.

- Eat only fruit for a day or two. Don't do this for more than two days and preferably only when you don't have to work or be too energetic. Afterwards, go back to Phase 2, Week 2 and continue as before.

- Check whether you are consuming lots of hidden carbohydrates. See page 182 for more information and make sure you cut them out so you get back to the carbohydrate level you really want.

- Go on a calorie-controlled phase for a week or two, then go back to the low-carbohydrate regime. Stick to 1,000–1,200 calories per day for a woman, 1,200–1,500 for a man (*The Hugely Better Carbohydrate Counter* will give you the calorie content of everything you want to eat). At the end of two weeks of calorie-counting, go back to Phase 2, Week 2 of your low-carbohydrate diet, then continue from there as before.

Do not be tempted to reduce the amount of allowed fruit and vegetables, protein and fats you are eating whilst staying on the low-carbohydrate diet. Contrary to what you might imagine, this will slow your metabolism right down so you don't lose weight at all – and you won't be getting the nutrients you need either.

Slipping back

Because you can now have 'treats', it is very easy to think 'An extra bar of chocolate won't hurt' – and on its own, it probably won't. The trouble is, before you know it, this will become a habit, and you'll have started eating cakes, chocolates, sweet, sugary desserts – the lot! Having trained your body so well for so long, you shouldn't throw it all away now. Remember, treats really should be treats and that means only a couple of times a week.

The treats

Your treats are all laid out in the diet plan so, providing you follow it, you can't go wrong. You'll see that some of them are highly nutritious, but many are purely for indulgence. They all have 15 g of carbs, or fewer. If you find you start to gain weight with this level of 'treats', cut them back again. It's up to you to manage your body according to its metabolism.

You can put two 'treats' together in one meal, such as a slice of toast with butter **and** marmalade, but make sure you remember that you've had two-in-one!

Two or three times a week add any of the following:

- 100 g/4 oz new or old potatoes, steamed, boiled or mashed (with butter or margarine, if liked) or a **small** jacket-baked potato (with butter or margarine, grated cheese, crème fraîche and chive dressing or mayonnaise)

- A generous portion of crispy potato skins
  Scrub your potatoes before peeling them in the usual way. Put the peelings on a baking (cookie) sheet and bake in a hot oven at 200°C/400°F/gas 6/fan oven 180°C for about 20 minutes until crisp and golden. Season lightly with salt and pepper and leave to cool. Store them in an airtight container for a few days, if necessary. Enjoy for a delicious, nutritious snack (only 7 g of carbohydrates per medium potato, so you can have up to 2 medium potatoes-worth per serving!).
  Note: Peeled potatoes can also be stored covered with water in an airtight container in the fridge for up to 24 hours. Drain and cook in fresh water.

- 1 thin slice of bread (preferably wholemeal), from a large sliced loaf, with butter, if liked

- 1 medium slice of an uncut loaf, such as a bloomer, with butter, if liked

- 1 slice of currant bread, with butter, if liked

- 1 crumpet, with butter or margarine, if liked

- A portion of gnocchi, with butter and Parmesan cheese, if liked
- 2 small slices of garlic bread
- 1 individual Yorkshire pudding
- 1 Weetabix or Shredded Wheat, with unsweetened fortified soya milk
- 2 heaped tbsp cooked couscous or bulghar (cracked wheat)
- 3 heaped tbsp cooked dried peas, beans or lentils
- 2 plain biscuits (cookies) or 1 biscuit half-coated in chocolate
- 2 sponge (lady) fingers
- ½ standard bar of chocolate or 1 fun-size bar
- 1 scoop of ice-cream
- 1 tbsp (2 tbsp if reduced-sugar) jam (conserve), marmalade or honey
- 1 small bag of potato crisps (chips)
- 1 onion bhaji or pakora
- 2 poppadoms
- 1 small pancake roll
- 1 meat samosa
- 1 potato waffle
- 1 hash brown
- 5 deep-fried onion rings
- 1 pancake, with lemon and sugar
- 1 pint of beer
- ½ pint of medium-sweet cider
- 1 double measure (50 ml) of sweet vermouth or sherry
- 2 glasses of Sangria
- 1 lemonade shandy
- 1 sweetened speciality coffee, such as Gaelic coffee

Phase 4: Maintaining the New You

Congratulations! You've reached your target! Now is the time to start eating sensibly – for ever. Don't worry, though: that doesn't mean never having favourite foods like chips (fries), pasta or chocolate. It just means eating them in moderation, along with fairly high-protein, low-carbohydrate meals, so that your diet will always give you a good balance of nutrients. You can maintain your weight, and at the same time shape your diet to include almost everything you may want to eat.

You can have any grilled (broiled), fried, poached or roasted meat, fish or poultry and any cheeses you like and most vegetables and fruits. You can also have cereals, such as oats and wheat, and bread, pasta, etc. I would recommend that you eat whole grains, but I know that these are not very popular and in reality, good-quality white products are okay. Just don't overdo those starchy foods and keep processed sugars – such as biscuits (cookies), cakes and sweets (candies) – for special treats. They should never form part of your everyday eating, as they can undo all your good work very quickly.

It is a good idea to keep a record of the amount of carbohydrate you are eating every day as well as continuing to weigh yourself every week, so that you will be able to see exactly what level will keep your weight constant.

Make a note of any weight you put on or lose. This is very important, so that you can act quickly if you find you are gaining weight. If this happens, you must cut back on the carbohydrates – particularly the 'treats'. Never cut out the low-carbohydrate vegetables and fruit (listed in Phases 1 and 2): these are vital for good health. But remember too, that when you start to include a reasonable quantity of carbohydrates, you will probably need to cut back on the fats – so don't have too much butter, cream, crème fraîche or fatty meats, like salami, or too many fried (sautéed) foods.

Watch points
OVEREATING
As I've said before, long term you should be eating a balanced diet, including nutrients from all the food groups. Now that you are eating a reasonable quantity of carbohydrates, make sure you don't eat an excessive quantity of proteins and fats too. If you do, you will be consuming too much food in undesirable quantities.

Watch your intake of calories as well as carbohydrates. Your daily calorie total should be no more than 2,000 calories a day for a woman, 2,500 calories a day for a man. Aim for a balanced diet, that includes the following every day:

- Plenty of low-carb fruit and vegetables
- 2–3 portions of protein
- A reasonable amount of starchy carbohydrates
- Very little added sugar
- Very little added fat

HIDDEN CARBOHYDRATES
We all know that carbohydrates are contained in starchy foods like bread, pasta, rice and potatoes, and that sugars are found in sweet things like fruit, cakes, chocolate, biscuits, sweets (candies) and ice cream. But carbohydrates are found in lots of other foods that may surprise you. Always read the labels when shopping so that you can make informed choices. Most important, be wary of any food that claims to be 'low-fat' or 'light': these will nearly always have **added** starches or sugars to compensate for the reduced amount of fat.

Check out the following:

Meats, seafood and poultry

- Some delicatessen meats
- Processed meat products, like sausages, frankfurters, pâtés and potted meats
- Crab sticks and other imitation fish products
- Fish fingers and pastes; canned fish in sauce
- Shaped chicken and turkey fingers, drumsticks, etc.

Remember some offal and fish contain small amounts of carbohydrates naturally.

Dairy products

- Milk
- Yoghurts (especially the low-fat and fat-free thick ones, which have starchy fillers)
- Cheese spread
- Dried milk (non-fat dry milk)

Note that fresh, soft cheeses have more carbohydrates in the lower-fat versions.

Sauces, dressings and condiments

Many have sugar and/or starch added. You may expect these in pickles and chutneys, but they turn up in some unexpected places, so read the labels on everything, including the following:

- Tomato ketchup (catsup)
- Commercial salad cream
- Bought French dressing
- Blended spices and baking powder, which may contain starchy fillers
- Garlic purée (paste)
- Speciality vinegars
- Mustards
- Soy sauce

- Coffee whitener
- Stock cubes

Drinks

- Coffee and cocoa contain some carbohydrates.
- Beers, sweet wines and liqueurs have lots.
- Watch out for diet drinks. Unless they are labelled as containing 0 calories, they will, probably, contain some carbs. Always check the labels and be sensible. You will note that a few recipes I have called for sugar-free real blackcurrant cordial. Undiluted, it has 0.5 g carbohydrates per 30 ml/2 tbsp, so a tablespoonful isn't going to make much difference to your carbohydrate intake in a day. But, if you were to drink, say, 10 small glasses in a day, that would be an extra 5 g of carbohydrates. And if you had large glasses, it could amount to as much as 10 g!

REGULAR EXERCISE

Exercise is vital to stimulate metabolism. An active body is more likely to be a healthy body. One mad burst a week at the gym isn't a good idea. You need to go more frequently to reap the benefit, and so this is only going to be a success if you like that sort of thing. But there are plenty of other ways to get regular exercise without jogging or work-outs.

- Walk briskly instead of strolling.
- Walk whenever possible instead of using the car or public transport.
- If you take the bus, get off a stop before your usual one and walk the last part of the journey.
- Ride a bike if you have one.
- Use stairs instead of lifts or escalators.
- Take up a recreational sport, such as tennis or swimming, or join a dance class. Even gardening will burn off calories, especially if you are digging or doing other energetic tasks.
- Bending and stretching exercises will also help to tone your muscles but you must do them properly or you could cause an injury. Seek advice before you start. If you are going to

do this at home, make the exercises a regular part of your daily routine, perhaps as soon as you get out of bed or before you have your shower or bath in the morning or evening. If you don't, the novelty will wear off after a few days and you won't persevere.

Meal Planning
BREAKFAST
Vary what you have for breakfast each day. You can choose a high-protein breakfast two or three times a week (see any of the suggestions in this book), and on other days have a small bowl of your favourite cereal (preferably an unsweetened one), with cows' or unsweetened fortified soya milk according to your carbohydrate tolerance.

LUNCH
If you aren't having your main meal at lunchtime, go for a high-protein snack, such as a ham, egg, or tuna salad. Alternatively, try an avocado filled with prawns, cottage cheese or chopped bacon; or have some pâté or cheese, preferably with crispbreads rather than bread (or limit it to one slice) and a side salad. If you want something hot, choose from soup, an omelette or cheese fondue, with breadsticks or crudités rather than cubes of French bread, except on special occasions. Although don't have more than four eggs a week now – preferably fewer – they're high in cholesterol.

DINNER
You will probably find that if you reduce your fat content now – by cutting down on butter, cream, crème fraîche and higher fat meats, like salami, and foods cooked in fat or oil – you will be able to tolerate a reasonable amount of carbohydrate without gaining weight.

All of the recipes on the following pages include a small high-carbohydrate accompaniment. But you can also use any of the other recipes in this book and add a small portion of rice, pasta, couscous or potatoes.

Carbohydrate accompaniments

The portion size here is about half the average serving when on a normal mixed diet. This should be adequate for most people but by all means increase the quantities if you can tolerate them without gaining weight. It's up to you to manage your diet to match your lifestyle and your body.

Item	Serving size	Carbs per serving
Long-grain rice	About 2 heaped tbsp cooked (25 g/1 oz uncooked)	28 g
Bulghar (cracked wheat)	About 2 heaped tbsp cooked (25 g/1 oz uncooked)	14 g
Couscous	About 2 heaped tbsp cooked (25 g/1 oz uncooked)	14 g
Pasta	About 2 heaped tbsp cooked (40 g/1½ oz uncooked)	21 g
Home-made chips (fries) or sautéed potatoes	1 medium potato	25 g
Fries from burger outlet	Small portion	28 g

Desserts

Take care when choosing desserts. Use any in this book, or have fresh fruit on its own or as a fruit salad in natural juice. If buying individual ready-made desserts, remember that low-sugar ones tend to have fewer carbohydrates (check the labels), whereas low-fat ones aren't good low-carbohydrate options as they often contain extra sugars. Have sweet, sticky puddings only on special occasions and, if possible, only when you've had a low-carbohydrate main course. If you really must indulge, remember that the smaller the portion is, the fewer the carbohydrates! Finally, if you've already blown out on a stodgy starter and main course, have cheese instead of a dessert, but go steady on the biscuits (crackers) or bread!

Main Meal Recipes

These are main-meal recipes that all the family can enjoy. While they eat everything, you can omit the added higher-carbohydrate extras if you find you start to gain weight again. Many of the main dishes, such as Tandoori Chicken, contain no carbs at all. It's up to you to manage your body and your eating habits.

You can, of course, use any of the recipes from other chapters of this book. If you use the ones from Phases 1 and 2, you can 'top them up' by adding an accompaniment of a little bread, pasta, rice, couscous, etc., or higher-carbohydrate vegetables or fruits, such as a potato or banana. As ever, balance is the key.

All these recipes serve four people, so that you can share them with friends or family, or they can be divided to make one or two portions as necessary.

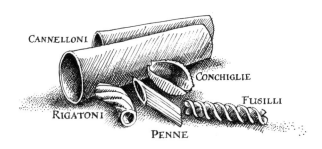

CANNELLONI · CONCHIGLIE · FUSILLI · RIGATONI · PENNE

Lamb tagine with pine nut couscous

An exotic Moroccan blend of tender lamb with apricots and vegetables bathed in a sweet spicy sauce on a bed of couscous, dotted with toasted pine nuts and fragrant fresh coriander.

700 g/1½ lb diced stewing lamb

5 ml/1 tsp ground cinnamon

5 ml/1 tsp ground ginger

5 ml/1 tsp ground cumin

2.5 ml/½ tsp salt

1 garlic clove, crushed

Freshly ground black pepper

45 ml/3 tbsp olive oil

1 onion, chopped

2 courgettes (zucchini), sliced

1 yellow or orange (bell) pepper, diced

100 g/4 oz/⅔ cup ready-to-eat dried apricots, quartered

600 ml/1 pt/2½ cups lamb or vegetable stock, made with 1 stock cube

30 ml/2 tbsp tomato purée (paste)

10 ml/2 tsp artificial sweetener

1 Mix the meat with all the spices, the salt, garlic and a good grinding of pepper. Toss with your hands to coat completely.

2 Heat 15 ml/1 tbsp of the oil in a flameproof casserole dish (Dutch oven). Add the onion, courgettes and pepper and stir-fry for 2 minutes. Remove from the casserole with a draining spoon and reserve.

3 Heat the remaining oil in the casserole, add the meat and brown all over, stirring and turning the pieces as necessary.

4 Return the onion mixture to the pan and stir in the apricots, stock, tomato purée and sweetener. Bring to the boil, cover and simmer gently for 1½–2 hours until the meat is really tender. Taste and re-season if necessary.

5 Meanwhile, put the couscous in a bowl and cover with the boiling water and a good pinch of salt. Stir and leave to stand for at least 5 minutes to swell. Fluff up with a fork.

6 Dry-fry the pine nuts in a frying pan (skillet) until golden. Stir into the couscous with half the coriander.

7 Sprinkle the tagine with the remaining coriander and serve with the couscous.

100 g/4 oz/²⁄₃ cup couscous

300 ml/½ pt/1¼ cups boiling water

60 ml/4 tbsp pine nuts

30 ml/2 tbsp chopped fresh coriander (cilantro)

Serves 4

Carbohydrates: 49 g per serving (including 32 g for the couscous)

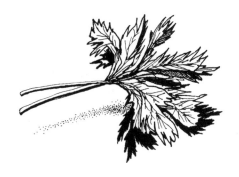

Trout with almonds and fresh parsley

A classic that can't be bettered: fresh trout, lightly cooked in olive oil and butter, topped with flaked almonds and fresh parsley, served with mangetout and garlic-flavoured sautéed potatoes.

For the potatoes:

4 medium potatoes, diced

Oil, for shallow-frying

1 large garlic clove, quartered

For the fish:

4 trout, cleaned

4 sprigs of thyme

45 ml/3 tbsp olive oil

25 g/1 oz/2 tbsp butter

Freshly ground black pepper

60 ml/4 tbsp flaked (slivered) almonds

15 ml/1 tbsp lemon juice

30 ml/2 tbsp chopped fresh parsley

Serve with:

200 g/7 oz mangetout (snow peas), steamed

Serves 4

Carbohydrates: 29 g per serving (27 g for the potatoes and 2 g for the mangetout)

1 Dry the potatoes well in a clean tea towel (dishcloth) or kitchen paper (paper towels).

2 Heat about 2.5 cm/1 in of oil in a heavy-based frying pan (skillet). Add the potatoes and garlic and fry (sauté) for about 6 minutes, stirring and turning occasionally, until golden brown all over. Drain on kitchen paper, discarding the pieces of garlic, and keep the potatoes warm.

3 Meanwhile, wipe the fish and cut the heads off, if liked. Push a sprig of thyme inside each one.

4 Heat the olive oil and butter in a large frying pan. Add the fish and add a good grinding of pepper. Fry for 4 minutes on each side until golden brown and cooked through. Carefully lift out of the pan on to warm plates and keep warm.

5 Add the nuts to the juices in the pan and fry, stirring, for about a minute until lightly browned. Add the lemon juice and parsley. Spoon over the fish and serve with the sautéed potatoes and mangetout.

Speciality seafood pie with white wine

In this elegant pie, the seafood is cooked in a delicious white wine and tomato sauce, then topped with buttery crumpled filo, baked until crisp.

1 Melt the butter in a saucepan, pour off half and reserve. Add the oil, leeks and garlic and cook gently, stirring, for 3 minutes until soft but not brown.

2 Skin and chop the tomatoes and add to the pan with the sweetener, wine and stock. Bring to the boil and cook for 5 minutes.

3 Gently stir in the seafood and cod, bring back to the boil, reduce the heat and cook gently for about 5 minutes until the fish is cooked but still holds its shape. Season to taste and stir in the crème fraîche and half the parsley.

4 Brush the remaining butter over a baking (cookie) sheet and the filo sheets, then gently scrunch each filo sheet like crumpled paper. Place on the baking sheet. Bake in a preheated oven at 190°C/375°F/gas 5/fan oven 170°C for 5 minutes until crisp and golden.

5 Meanwhile, steam or boil the mangetout and corn cobs.

6 Spoon the fish mixture on warm plates and top with the crumpled filo. Dust the edges of the plates with the remaining parsley and serve with the mangetout and baby corn cobs.

50 g/2 oz/¼ cup butter
15 ml/1 tbsp olive oil
2 leeks, cut into chunks
1 garlic clove, crushed
2 beefsteak tomatoes
2.5 ml/½ tsp artificial sweetener
150 ml/¼ pt/⅔ cup dry white wine
150 ml/¼ pt/⅔ cup fish stock
450 g/1 lb mixed seafood cocktail
225 g/8 oz cod fillet, skinned and diced
Salt and pepper
90 ml/6 tbsp crème fraîche
30 ml/2 tbsp chopped fresh parsley
4 large sheets of filo pastry (paste)
Serve with:
200 g/7 oz mangetout and 16 baby corn cobs

Serves 4

Carbohydrates: 20 g per serving (including 10 g for the topping and 5 g for the veg)

Choucroute garni with mustard mash

Sauerkraut, a popular German dish, is fermented cabbage with a unique flavour. Married with robust meats like belly pork and smoked sausage, it makes a hearty and tasty dish to enjoy.

15 ml/1 tbsp sunflower oil

1 medium onion, thinly sliced

1 x 700 g/1½ lb/large jar of sauerkraut, drained

A good pinch of ground cloves

1 bay leaf

4 rashers (slices) of belly pork

2 bacon chops, halved

1 smoked pork ring, cut into 8 chunks

150 ml/¼ pt/⅔ cup dry white wine

150 ml/¼ pt/⅔ cup chicken stock, made with ½ stock cube

Salt and freshly ground black pepper

For the mash:

450 g/1 lb potatoes, cut into small chunks

15 ml/1 tbsp grainy mustard

15 ml/1 tbsp chopped fresh parsley

1 Heat the oil in a large flameproof casserole dish (Dutch oven). Add the onion and fry (sauté) gently for 2 minutes, stirring, until softened but not browned.

2 Add the sauerkraut and cloves and stir gently until well mixed.

3 Add the bay leaf and all the meats, then pour over the wine and stock. Add a good grinding of pepper but no salt at this stage. Bring to the boil, cover with a well-buttered piece of greaseproof (waxed) paper that fits snugly on top of the contents of the casserole, cover tightly with a lid and transfer to a preheated oven at 190°C/375°F/gas 5/fan oven 170°C for 30 minutes.

4 Reduce the heat to 160°C/ 325°F/gas 3/fan oven 145°C and cook for a further 2 hours, checking after every 30 minutes and adding a little water, if necessary, to prevent the mixture drying out. The meats should all be very tender and moist.

5 About 30 minutes before the choucroute will be ready, boil the potatoes in lightly salted water until tender. Drain thoroughly and return to the pan. Heat over a low heat for a few minutes to dry out, stirring all the time, then mash thoroughly with the mustard, parsley and butter.

6 Discard the paper and bay leaf from the choucroute, then lift out the meats carefully, so they don't disintegrate. Taste the sauerkraut and add some salt and more pepper, if necessary. Spoon the sauerkraut on to warm plates and add the meats. Spoon the mash to one side.

7 Garnish the plates with sprigs of parsley and serve.

15 g/½ oz/1 tbsp butter
Sprigs of fresh parsley, for garnishing

Serves 4
Carbohydrates: 22 g per serving (including 15 g for the mash)

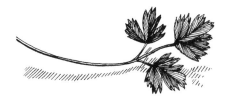

Low-carbohydrate lasagne verde

You don't have to miss out! This gives you lots of meat and a layer of courgettes instead of some pasta. You can make a very low-carb version using Soya Crêpes (see page 163) instead of pasta.

2 courgettes (zucchini)

30 ml/2 tbsp sunflower oil

1 onion, finely chopped

1 garlic clove, crushed

450 g/1 lb minced (ground) beef

1 x 400 g/14 oz/large can of chopped tomatoes

45 ml/3 tbsp tomato purée (paste)

60 ml/4 tbsp red wine

60 ml/4 tbsp water

5 ml/1 tsp dried oregano

Salt and freshly ground black pepper

2.5 ml/½ tsp artificial sweetener

4 sheets of green lasagne

1 egg

60 ml/4 tbsp double (heavy) cream

100 g/4 oz/1 cup grated Cheddar cheese

Serve with:

1 Cut each courgette lengthways into three slices, then fry (sauté) in the sunflower oil for about 2 minutes on each side until lightly golden. Remove from the pan.

2 Put the onion, garlic and beef in a saucepan. Cook, stirring all the time, until the meat is no longer pink and all the grains are separate.

3 Add the tomatoes, tomato purée, wine, water, oregano, some salt and pepper and the sweetener. Bring to the boil, stirring, reduce the heat and simmer for 20 minutes until thick and rich.

4 Spread a little of the meat mixture over the base of a shallow, rectangular ovenproof dish. Cover with two sheets of lasagne.

5 Spoon half the remaining meat over, then add a layer of the courgette slices. Top with all of the remaining meat, then the remaining lasagne sheets.

6 Beat the egg with the cream and cheese and a little salt and pepper. Spoon this sauce over the lasagne. Bake in a preheated oven at 190°C/375°F/gas 5/fan oven 170°C for about 35 minutes until the lasagne is tender and the top is golden brown.

7 Serve hot, accompanied by a green salad.

A Green Salad (see page 65)

Serves 4

Carbohydrates: 16 g per serving (including 2 g for the salad)

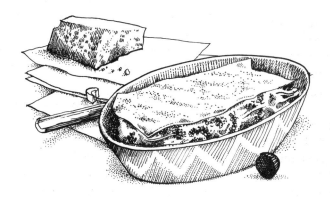

Roasted pork chops with a potato gratin

Thick, tender pork chops, cooked with olive oil and oregano, then laid on a bed of lightly cooked spinach leaves and served with a rich potato cake, baked in crème fraîche, cheese and garlic.

25 g/1 oz/2 tbsp butter

450 g/1 lb potatoes, scrubbed and sliced

1 garlic clove, crushed

Salt and freshly ground black pepper

100 g/4 oz/1 cup grated Gruyère (Swiss) cheese

2 eggs

150 ml/¹/₄ pt/²/₃ cup crème fraîche

150 ml/¹/₄ pt/²/₃ cup milk

4 pork chops, about 175 g/6 oz each

15 ml/1 tbsp olive oil

5 ml/1 tsp dried oregano

450 g/1 lb spinach, well-washed

300 ml/¹/₂ pt/1¹/₄ cups vegetable stock, made with 1 stock cube

1 Butter a fairly shallow ovenproof dish with half the butter.

2 Cook the sliced potatoes in boiling water for 3 minutes until just tender but still holding their shape. Drain well. Layer the potatoes in the dish with the garlic, some salt and pepper and the cheese, finishing with a layer of cheese.

3 Beat the eggs with the crème fraîche and milk. Pour over the potatoes.

4 Put the chops in a roasting tin (pan) and drizzle with the oil. Season the pork with a little salt and pepper, sprinkle on both sides with the oregano and dot with the remaining butter.

5 Put the potatoes towards the top of a preheated oven at 190°C/375°F/gas 5/fan oven 170°C and put the pork in the centre. Bake for 35 minutes, turning the chops over once halfway through cooking. The potatoes should be set and golden and the chops browned and cooked through.

6 Meanwhile, put the spinach in a saucepan and pour boiling water over it. Stir well, then leave to stand for 2 minutes, drain in a metal colander and keep warm. (You can set it over the pan with some hot water in it.)

7 Remove the cooked pork from the roasting tin. Add the vegetable stock to the pan and boil, scraping up any sediment, for a few minutes until reduced by half. Taste and re-season, if necessary.

8 Put the spinach on four plates. Put the chops on top and spoon the gravy over. Serve with the potatoes.

Serves 4

Carbohydrates: 21 g per serving (19 g for the potatoes and 2 g for the spinach)

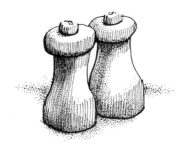

Herb-stuffed chicken breasts on risotto

Chicken breasts filled with herb butter in a golden almond and Parmesan coating. For each salad, lay a sliced tomato on a handful of rocket, drizzle with olive oil and balsamic vinegar.

50 g/2 oz/¼ cup butter, softened

15 ml/1 tbsp chopped fresh parsley

15 ml/1 tbsp chopped fresh thyme

5 ml/1 tsp chopped fresh sage

1.5 ml/¼ tsp celery salt

Freshly ground black pepper

30 ml/2 tbsp olive oil

4 part-boned chicken breasts, about 200 g/ 7 oz each

1 egg, beaten

60 ml/4 tbsp ground almonds

60 ml/4 tbsp grated Parmesan cheese

Sunflower oil, for cooking

For the risotto:

15 ml/1 tbsp olive oil

2 spring onions (scallions), finely chopped

225 g/8 oz button mushrooms, sliced

1 Mash the butter with the herbs, celery salt and a good grinding of pepper. Shape into a short, fat sausage on a piece of greaseproof (waxed) paper and roll up. Chill in the fridge until hard.

2 Make a slit in the side of each chicken breast. Cut the hardened butter into four pieces and push a piece in each pocket. Secure the slits with wooden cocktail sticks (toothpicks).

3 Beat the egg on a plate. Mix the nuts and cheese on another. Dip the chicken in the egg, then the nuts and cheese, to coat completely.

4 Heat 5 mm/¼ in of the oil in a non-stick frying pan (skillet). Add the chicken and fry (sauté) over a moderate heat for about 8 minutes on each side until golden brown and cooked through.

5 Meanwhile, make the risotto. Heat the oil in a saucepan, add the onion and mushrooms and cook, stirring, over a gentle heat for 2 minutes. Stir in the rice and cook for 30 seconds.

6 Add about a quarter of the stock and cook over a gentle heat, stirring occasionally until the rice has absorbed the liquid. Continue adding a little stock at a time until all is used. The rice should be just cooked and the risotto creamy. Season to taste.

7 Spoon the rice on to warm plates and arrange the chicken to one side. Remove the cocktail sticks.

8 Serve with a tomato and rocket salad.

100 g/4 oz/½ cup risotto rice

600 ml/1 pt/2½ cups hot vegetable stock, made with 1 stock cube

A little chopped fresh parsley, for garnishing

Serve with:

A dressed tomato and rocket salad

Serves 4

Carbohydrates: 32 g per serving (including 3 g for the salad)

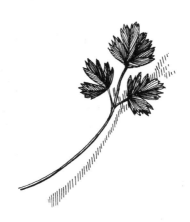

Tandoori chicken with dhal and salad

Rich, red, mildly spiced, marinated chicken baked until tinged black on the outside but juicy and succulent inside, served with a fragrant spicy lentil dhal and a crisp, cool salad.

2 small chickens, each about 1.25 kg/2½ lb, or 4 large chicken portions

Juice of 1 lime or small lemon

2.5 ml/½ tsp each of red and yellow food colouring

300 ml/½ pt/1¼ cups plain Greek-style strained cows' milk yoghurt

1 small garlic clove, crushed

2.5 ml/½ tsp ground ginger

15 ml/1 tbsp garam masala

15 ml/1 tbsp paprika

1.5 ml/¼ tsp chilli powder

1 Pull off as much of the skin from the chickens as possible. Cut into quarters and make several slashes in the flesh.

2 Mix the lime or lemon juice with the food colourings and brush all over the chicken.

3 Mix the yoghurt with the garlic and spices in a large roasting tin (pan). Add the chicken pieces and turn over in the mixture to coat completely, rubbing it well into the slits. Cover and leave to marinate for at least 3 hours, turning at least once.

4 Arrange the chicken pieces, flesh-sides down and transfer the roasting tin to the oven preheated at 200°C/ 400°F/gas 6/fan oven 180°C. Cook for 20 minutes, then drain off any liquid. Turn the chicken over and cook for a further 20 minutes.

5 Meanwhile, make the dahl. Put the lentils, water, spices, a good pinch of salt and a generous grinding of black pepper in a saucepan. Bring to the boil, reduce the heat and simmer for about 20 minutes until pulpy.

6 Fry (sauté) the onion in the oil for 2 minutes. Add the ginger and chilli and fry for a further 2 minutes until golden. Add to the dhal with the tomato, cover and cook for a further 10 minutes, stirring occasionally.

7 Serve the chicken with the dhal and a side salad of the lettuce, tomatoes and cucumber, garnished with wedges of lemon and sprigs of coriander.

For the dhal:

225 g/8 oz/1⅓ cups red lentils

900 ml/1½ pts/3¾ cups water

2.5 ml/½ tsp ground turmeric

4 split cardamom pods

1 piece of cinnamon stick

2 cloves

Salt and freshly ground black pepper

1 onion, thinly sliced

30 ml/2 tbsp oil

5 ml/1 tsp grated fresh root ginger

1 green chilli, seeded and finely chopped

1 tomato, skinned and chopped

For the side salad:

4 wedges of lettuce, shredded

4 tomatoes, quartered

10 cm/4 in piece of cucumber, sliced

Wedges of lemon and sprigs of fresh coriander (cilantro)

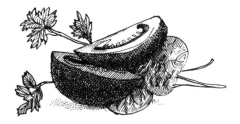

Serves 4

Carbohydrates: 28 g per serving 20 g for the dhal and 8 g for the salad)

Chinese chicken and cashew nuts with seaweed

Cashew nuts with chicken mingle here with spring onions, carrot and beansprouts in a lightly thickened soy-flavoured sauce, served with crispy 'seaweed' and oriental-style fried rice.

100 g/4 oz/½ cup long-grain rice

50 g/2 oz/½ cup frozen peas

45 ml/3 tbsp sunflower oil

A good pinch of Chinese five-spice powder

2 eggs, beaten

450 g/1 lb boneless chicken thighs, skinned and cut into neat strips

1 bunch of spring onions (scallions), cut diagonally into short lengths

1 carrot, grated

225 g/8 oz/4 cups beansprouts

100 g/4 oz/1 cup raw cashew nuts

300 ml/½ pt/1¼ cups chicken stock, made with 1 stock cube

10 ml/2 tsp arrowroot

15 ml/1 tbsp soy sauce

Oil, for deep-frying

1 Cook the rice in plenty of boiling, lightly salted water for 10 minutes, adding the peas after 5 minutes. Drain thoroughly.

2 Heat 15 ml/1 tbsp of the oil in a frying pan (skillet). Add the rice and stir until every grain is glistening. Push the rice to one side of the pan and sprinkle with the five-spice powder. Tilt the pan and add the eggs. Gradually draw the egg into the rice a little at a time as it cooks, so that it forms strands in the rice. When all the egg is cooked, remove the pan from the heat, ready to reheat just before serving.

3 Heat the remaining oil in a large frying pan or wok. Add the chicken and stir-fry for 2 minutes.

4 Add the spring onions and stir-fry for a further 2 minutes. Add the carrot, beansprouts, nuts and stock. Bring to the boil, reduce the heat and simmer for 5 minutes, stirring occasionally. Blend the arrowroot with the soy sauce and stir in. Boil for 1 minute until thickened.

5 Meanwhile, heat the oil for deep-frying until a cube of day-old bread browns in 30 seconds. Deep-fry the shredded greens in batches for 2 minutes until crispy. Drain each batch on kitchen paper (paper towels).

6 Reheat the rice. Spoon on to warm plates with the chicken and pile the seaweed to one side. Sprinkle with the sesame seeds and serve.

350 g/12 oz spring (collard) greens, finely shredded

30 ml/2 tbsp sesame seeds

Serves 4

Carbohydrates: 43 g per serving (including 29 g for the rice and 3 g for the seaweed)

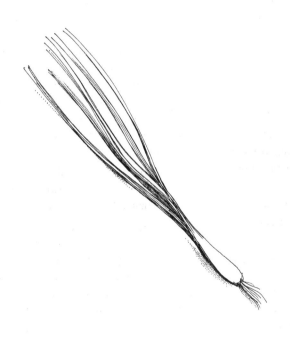

Beef in red wine
with baby jacket potatoes

Lean, tender diced steak slowly cooked in red wine with lardons, herbs, garlic and vegetables until meltingly tender, complemented with baby baked potatoes.

700 g/1½ lb braising steak, diced

50 g/2 oz lardons (diced bacon)

1 red onion, chopped

1 garlic clove, crushed

1 carrot, sliced

225 g/8 oz baby button mushrooms

300 ml/½ pt/1¼ cups red wine

150 ml/¼ pt/⅔ cup beef stock made with ½ a stock cube

15 ml/1 tbsp tomato purée (paste)

Salt and pepper

12 small potatoes

25 g/1 oz/2 tbsp butter

30 ml/2 tbsp snipped fresh chives

Serve with:

450 g/1 lb broccoli, steamed

Serves 4

Carbohydrates: 39 g per serving (including 32 g for the potatoes and 2g for broccoli)

1 Put all the ingredients except the potatoes, butter and chives in a flameproof casserole dish (Dutch oven). Bring to the boil. Cover with a lid and transfer to a preheated oven at 150°C/300°F/gas 2/fan oven 135°C for 3½ hours.

2 After 2 hours, melt the butter in a baking tin (pan). Add the potatoes and roll them in the butter. Bake at the top of the oven with the beef, turning the potatoes once, until everything is tender.

3 Stir the casserole, taste and re-season if necessary. Sprinkle the potatoes with the chives and serve with the casserole and broccoli.

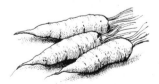

Index